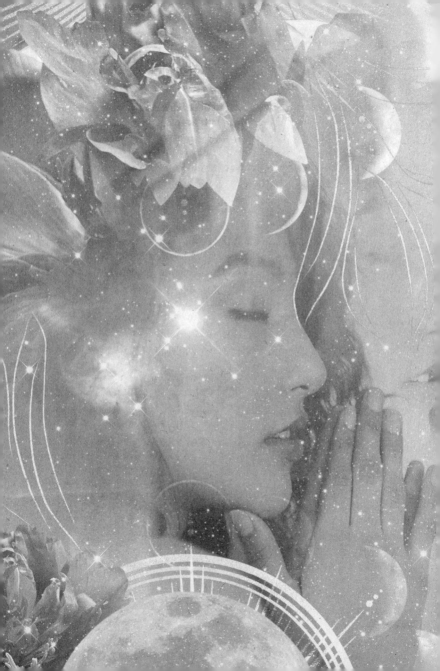

365
HAPPY
BEDTIME
MANTRAS

IMPROVE YOUR SLEEP, RELEASE STRESS,
ENJOY YOUR DREAMS

SHANNON KAISER

ATRIA PAPERBACK
New York Amsterdam/Antwerp London
Toronto Sydney/Melbourne New Delhi

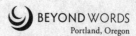
BEYOND WORDS
Portland, Oregon

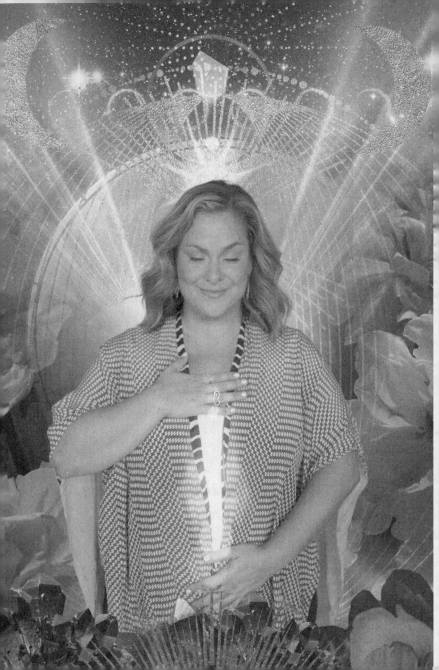

Also by Shannon Kaiser

BOOKS

Return to You: 11 Spiritual Lessons for Unshakable Inner Peace

Joy Seeker: Let Go of What's Holding You Back So You Can Live the Life You Were Made For

The Self-Love Experiment: 15 Principles for Becoming More Kind, Compassionate, and Accepting of Yourself

Adventures for Your Soul: 21 Ways to Transform Your Habits and Reach Your Full Potential

Find Your Happy Daily Mantras: 365 Days of Motivation for a Happy, Peaceful, and Fulfilling Life

OTHER DECKS

Happy Bedtime Mantras Card Deck: Improve Your Sleep, Release Stress, and Enjoy Your Dreams

Guidance from Gaia Oracle: Practices and Affirmations from Spirit Animals

Unshakable Inner Peace Oracle Cards: A 44-Card Deck and Guidebook to Awaken & Align with Your True Power

Find Your Happy Daily Mantra Deck

ATRIA PAPERBACK
An Imprint of Simon & Schuster, Inc.
1230 Avenue of the Americas
New York, NY 10020

BEYOND WORDS
1750 S.W. Skyline Blvd., Suite 20
Portland, Oregon 97221-2543
503-531-8700 / 503-531-8773 fax
www.beyondword.com

Managing editor: Lindsay Easterbrooks-Brown
Editors: Michele Ashtiani Cohn, Bailey Potter
Copyeditor: Jennifer Weaver-Neist
Proofreader: Ashley Van Winkle
Illustrations: Shannon Kaiser
Design: Sara E. Blum
Composition: William H. Brunson Typography Services

This first Beyond Words/Atria Paperback edition March 2025

ATRIA PAPERBACK and colophon are trademarks of Simon & Schuster, LLC.

BEYOND WORDS PUBLISHING is an imprint of Simon & Schuster, LLC, and the Beyond Words logo is a registered trademark of Beyond Words Publishing, Inc.

For information about special discounts for bulk purchases, please contact Simon & Schuster Special Sales at 1-866-506-1949 or business@simonandschuster.com.

The Simon & Schuster Speakers Bureau can bring authors to your live event. For more information or to book an event, contact the Simon & Schuster Speakers Bureau at 1-866-248-3049 or visit our website at www.simonspeakers.com.

Manufactured in the USA

10 9 8 7 6 5 4 3 2 1

Library of Congress Control Number: 2024050612

The corporate mission of Beyond Words Publishing, Inc.: *Inspire to Integrity*

To my brother, Clint,
the most peaceful, calm, and kindest person I know.
Love you.

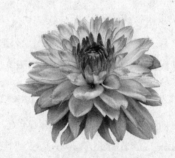

CONTENTS

THE BEDTIME MANTRAS

1: Bedtime Mantras for Relaxation

2: BEDTIME MANTRAS FOR RELEASING STRESS

3: Bedtime Mantras for Enjoying Dreams

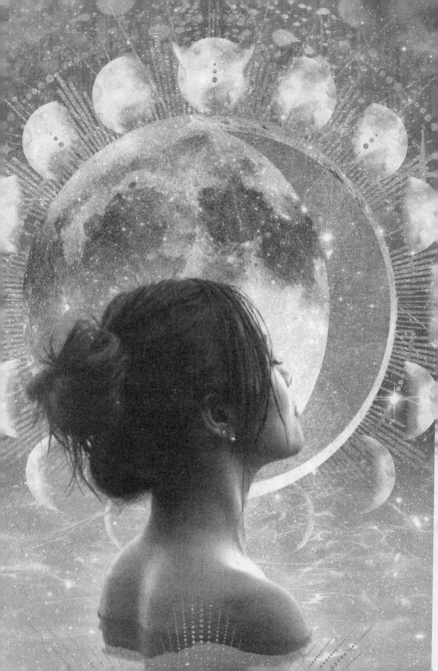

PREFACE

When is the last time you had a wonderful night's sleep? Most of us would call ourselves lucky if we could fall asleep easily, sleep soundly through the night, experience and remember our dreams, and wake up feeling refreshed. But for one in three adults in the US (about eighty-four million people), experiencing uninterrupted sleep and getting a great night's rest is just a dream. The reality is sleep makes up one-third of our life (a good twenty-five to thirty years), and it impacts everything we do.[1] I know firsthand the impact of poor sleep and how it can cause mental stress and break down the body.

For years, I experienced brain fog, exhaustion, widespread pain, weight gain, insomnia, and multiple other health issues connected to sleep disruptions. It wasn't until I met with an internal medicine doctor who specialized in chronic illnesses as well as mind-body-spirit wellness that I started to see the connection between mental and physical health and how the quality of sleep—or lack thereof—impacts everything. After years of feeling dismissed, unseen, and gaslit by my regular doctor, it was a huge relief to meet with a health team that looked at the multiple layers of the problems, including lifestyle, diet, genetics, personal relationships, family history, and life stresses that could be affecting my mental health. This whole mind–body approach to wellness was a breakthrough that led me to do a sleep study, which gave the official diagnosis of severe sleep apnea. That is when I realized how important sleep is to our overall health—that prioritizing rest is *essential* to our well-being.

Sleep apnea is a common condition in which your breathing stops and restarts many times while you sleep, preventing the body from getting enough oxygen. It is just one of several sleep disorders that are running rampant in today's world—roughly thirty-nine million adults in the US have sleep apnea.[2] But whether you have difficulty falling asleep or staying asleep, have experienced other sleep disturbances, or simply want to feel more energy during the day because your body and mind are well rested, one thing is certain: better sleep creates a higher quality of life.

To live well means we must focus on sleeping well. Subtle shifts, one evening at a time, can reap tremendous rewards for your overall well-being. Understanding how one area of our life could be impacting another, and that everything is connected, the whole mind–body approach to wellness is the foundation for the process in this book.

You hold in your hands a guide to feeling better from the inside out. Each day is like a mini, personalized plan that addresses the ways in which different areas of your well-being could be impacting one another, as well as key health basics like nutrition, movement, somatic and healing exercises, stress management, breathwork, and mindfulness techniques for mind-body-spirit balance. This book is full of sleep optimization solutions to help you live well morning and night.

As someone who was diagnosed with clinical depression and crippling anxiety several years ago, I know how important it is to have tools and routines established to soothe our mind and body. I've managed to overcome my anxiety and depression and other mental health ailments with lifestyle changes and daily rituals—I did a deep dive into my own personal care routine, studying ways of bringing these same tools into my sleep process.

Knowing that there is never a one-size-fits-all method (everybody has different needs and processes), you'll find a variety of sleep solutions. What I have learned, however, is that some signature remedies are go-tos recommended by wise sages, mystics, and leaders, no matter what area of your life is affected. The act of doing rituals has been scientifically shown to reduce anxiety and improve performance, elevating our daily experience overall.[3] It wasn't until I established a bedtime routine that included these mindfulness, stress-relief, and body-balancing tools that I started to find a more consistent restful state. The results were amazing! I began to feel less stressed, I was more empowered throughout the day, and best of all, I reconnected to my dreams. Not only did my sleep improve but my health did too, which was reflected in my bloodwork, with biomarkers reading biologically younger. When we sleep well, our body repairs well, restoring itself from the demands and stresses of the day.

Much of my professional work over the past fourteen years has been focused on mental health, psychology, and spirituality, and how these impact our overall well-being. In combining these sectors, I have learned a delicate balance where science meets grace and wisdom fuels experiments—I think we all need to approach our wellness in this manner. As a mindset coach, I have seen clients continue to express their enthusiasm for mantras and tools to help them feel better each day. A few years before I wrote this book, I trained in functional nutrition and took the twenty-week, two-hundred-hour mindbodygreen health-coaching training, which included an overview on the effects of sleep on our lives. In this book, I combine all of these layers with the valuable insights from my own life experience. I've been teaching these tools to sold-out international retreats and wellness workshops, as well as to individual clients; *Spirituality & Health* magazine even dubbed me the "Mantra Girl"! Kind of fun, right?

We all have the power to feel better, and you can be your own mantra queen or king. It starts with the simple steps we take each day and night. Small lifestyle tweaks like those that I recommend in this book help to transition our waking body, mind, and spirit into deep relaxation and rest when we sleep. When I started to share these methods with retreat participants and coaching clients, the impact it had on their

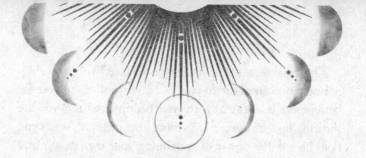

overall health and wellness was undeniable. People told me how they felt more energized and focused during the day; felt more self-love, confidence, and compassion; how they began looking forward to their evening routines again; how they were sleeping better, waking refreshed; and how they were better able to manage daily stress and anxiety.

I released *Find Your Happy Daily Mantras* in 2018, and clients and readers around the world still share how this book has transformed their lives. So, when my publisher came to me with the idea to write the book *365 Happy Bedtime Mantras* and the companion forty-four-card deck, *Happy Bedtime Mantras Card Deck*, it made complete sense—it was time to share these tools with even more people.

By practicing these tools and processes I share in this book, I am much more active and present, I feel better in my body, I sleep much more soundly at night, and I wake up earlier, looking forward to productive days. My bedtime-mantra routine is a large part of this successful transformation. By regaining my health, I was able to re-energize my entire life and focus on my dreams again, both at night and in my waking life. It even led me to move full-time to one of my favorite places on earth—Puerto Vallarta, Mexico—where I wrote this book.

This book is a gift of stress-free, relaxed living and sleep optimization from me to you, but also from *you* to you. By being more intentional with your bedtime routine, you are showing up for yourself with more love and care. What you hold here is the power of reclaiming your own power and energy. In the same way this practice has helped me, may you find lasting mental, spiritual, physical, and emotional peace as you enjoy 365 days of happy bedtime mantras.

With love,

Shannon Kaiser

INTRODUCTION

WE ALL NEED BETTER SLEEP

We all know getting a good night's sleep is important, but how many of us are prioritizing it and making it part of our wellness routine? In today's overstimulated, 24/7, always-connected, perpetually on-the-go conditioning of the world, millions are experiencing anxiety and sleep issues, including insomnia, snoring, restless leg syndrome, and sleep apnea. Sleep disorders impact fifty to seventy million Americans[4] and cost billions in medical expenses, accidents, and daily loss of productivity.[5] No matter how well you eat, how consistent you are with exercise, or how strong or smart you are, none of it will matter much if you're not sleeping and breathing properly.

And if we keep pushing past sleep disruptions and ignoring healthy wind-down routines, this will impact every other area of our lives.

Getting a good night's rest is not just about recharging the body but also resting our mind. As we are all exposed to collective trauma, environmental challenges, and fears in our daily lives, our minds work overtime to process the overwhelming world, and quality sleep becomes even more crucial—without it, our bodies start to break down. Unfortunately, daily stresses and demands take precedence for many, and prioritizing our bedtime routines has become the last things on our minds.

While more than half a million people in the US have been diagnosed with a sleep disorder, it's estimated that many more suffer but go undiagnosed and untreated.[6] This lack of sleep is degrading our health; we feel it in our energy levels (we have difficulty focusing), it can negatively affect our relationships[7], and it can even contribute to chronic illnesses.[8] Here are some more recent facts on the results of poor sleep in the US:

- about one in three adults reported not getting enough rest or sleep every day;[9]

- 54.4 percent of adults report stress and anxiety to be the top reasons they have trouble falling asleep;[10]

- 94.8 percent of adults lose at least an hour of sleep due to physical pain in a given week;[11]

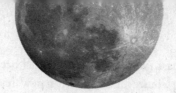

- 70 percent of adults report waking up tired;[12]

- 42 percent of adults begin feeling tired by noon;[13]

- 70 to 91 percent of adults with post-traumatic stress disorder (PTSD) experience difficulty falling or staying asleep;[14] and

- the US economy may lose as much as $411 billion per year due to insufficient sleep.[15]

On the flip side, science shows that reversing these negative effects can be as easy as prioritizing good sleep with consistent bedtime routines.[16]

It seems humanity is silently suffering emotionally, physically, and mentally in an epidemic of poor sleep. When I mention poor sleep, I am not just talking about insomnia, sleep apnea, snoring, etc.; two of the biggest impacts from the lack of quality sleep is a clouded mental landscape and exponentially diminished daily function. Essentially, stress is impacting how we show up in the world, how we relate to others, and our performance levels. Sleep represents an integral cornerstone of overall health and well-being. True, a balanced, whole-food, nutrition-focused diet and regular exercise are still essential foundations for good health, but the impact of quality sleep can no longer be dismissed.

Over the past twenty years, there has been a dedicated focus on the science of sleep, with new research sharing health-ensuring benefits. The good news is we have the power to shift this, through intention, ritual, mindfulness, and mantras. Some positive sleep advantages include boosting our cognitive brain function to help us learn, make smart choices, and strengthen our memory recall. Getting adequate sleep also helps us regulate and balance our body's hormones, gut biome, emotions, immune function, and cardiovascular system, lowering blood pressure and keeping our hearts healthy—and all while fine-tuning our cellular structure and metabolic function.[17] Emerging research even proves the profound benefits of dreaming. As I always say, our dreams are the signature to our own potential, and they guide us to understanding layers of our waking life by subconscious processing. Matthew Walker, sleep expert and author of *Why We Sleep: Unlocking the Power of Sleep and Dreams*, writes in his book, "Dreaming provides a . . . consoling neurochemical bath that mollifies painful memories and a virtual reality space in which the brain melds past and present knowledge, inspiring creativity."[18] It's obvious: without quality sleep, everything else inevitably suffers.

Fortunately, a variety of simple tweaks to our bedtime routine can relax our racing minds and overworked bodies, lulling us to sleep, increasing the mind-body-spirit connection, and supporting the quality of rest we receive each night, from the time before we get into bed until we wake up the next morning.

How to Get the Most Out of These Practices and Your Sleep

I organized the structure of this book to align with key attributes of a quality evening wind-down routine. We will be looking at all areas of your life, such as the quality of your relationships, your stress levels, as well as your sleep routine, because—let's face it—they're all connected. Lifestyle choices impact the way your body processes and assimilates the emotional, physical, and mental outlook you have on life, and this all affects your physical body.

Here are some key components to consider as you start to create your own evening wind-down routine.

LISTEN TO YOUR BODY

The same way you may take a nap when you need it, rest calls to you when your body is craving it. Start studying your body's cues for sleep so you can anticipate supporting its needs. Many experts say it is wise to go to bed at the same time every night, but I operate under a different process. My body tells me what it needs, and I honor it. It's good to listen to the experts, but you are your own best teacher, healer, and guru. In listening to my body, I tend to go to sleep about the same time each night, because this feels best for keeping up with all the work that I do (coaching,

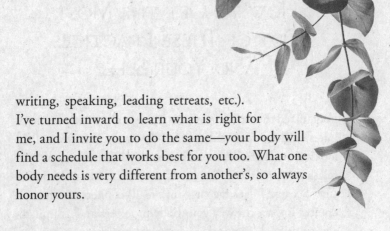

writing, speaking, leading retreats, etc.).
I've turned inward to learn what is right for
me, and I invite you to do the same—your body will
find a schedule that works best for you too. What one
body needs is very different from another's, so always
honor yours.

QUALITY OVER QUANTITY

We have all heard that a solid eight hours of sleep a night is
recommended, but the quality of sleep matters more than
anything. However, being in bed eight hours, tossing and
turning, and never reaching REM (restless eye movement,
aka the deepest stage of restful sleep) can wreak havoc on
the body and mind. Studies have shown that poor sleep
quality is significantly associated with higher stress levels
and mood disturbances.[19] Poor sleep can even predict lower
levels of exercise[20] and make it harder for us to feel productive and active during the day. Ideally, a night of quality
sleep means (1) you begin sleeping within twenty or so minutes of trying to sleep, (2) you spend about 85 percent of
your time in bed actually asleep,[21] (3) you don't wake up
during the night more than once or twice,[22] and (4) you
wake up feeling refreshed, or at least well rested.

How to
Use This Book

365 Happy Bedtime Mantras is a guide to help you feel better from the inside out all year long, at any time of the day, and especially at night. Part lifestyle coach, part ritual manual, and part self-care guide, each of the 365 nightly entries includes a main mantra message, a description that expands on the mantra's teachings, a mini meditation that activates the intention behind the mantra, and a mindfulness evening ritual to cultivate a calm state and balance the body, mind, and spirit.

MANTRAS

Mantras are a significant part of a good wellness routine and form the framework for this book. Mantras are like affirmations and intentions: they help to direct our focus. The gift of mantra is presence—the word *mantra* comes from two Sanskrit words: *man*, or "mind," and *tra*, which means "transport" or "vehicle." You can think of mantras like music to your mind, instruments for toning and balancing your mental landscape, especially when you want to make it easier to relax or to deepen your meditation.[23] In this book, I have written the mantras to target several categories of sleep quality (relaxation, releasing stress, and enjoying dreams) while elevating your evening ritual.

MEDITATIONS

We've all heard that meditation relieves mental stress, relaxes the body, and activates the parasympathetic nervous system (aka what allows your body to "rest and digest"),[24] but research has proven it plain and simple: meditation improves sleep quality.[25] You'll find a meditation in every night's entry in italic type, written in first person to drop you deeper into your heart with each word in the passage. They are mini self-love practices to nurture your mind and body while authentically activating your mind-body-spirit connection.

RITUALS

A ritual is simply an established routine or a ceremony in which the actions and wording follow a prescribed form and order. Along with the daily mantras and meditations, each day has a wind-down ritual such as breathwork, journal prompts, and other practices for relieving stress and preparing for a better night's sleep.

. . . . ● ● ◉ ● ● . . . .

This book is set up to serve you in whatever way works best. You can read one mantra during the day and add its description, meditation, and ritual into that night's routine; you can wait until you're winding down for the evening to read the night's entry; or you can open the book to any page, at any time during the day or night, for a quick moment of stress relief and mindfulness.

Please note that the book and its companion, *Happy Bedtime Mantras Card Deck*, work best when you implement them into a nightly routine, ideally an hour or two before bed. It's also a good idea to keep a notebook on your nightstand or close to your bed, as there are opportunities to journal in many of the evening rituals. If you aren't a journaling type of person, you can simply think about or meditate on the journal prompts when offered. Again, make this practice your own, as you will be more likely to stick with it consistently and see results. (The next section, on page xxxix, offers more suggestions on what to include in a personalized sleep-wellness toolkit.)

I designed this book in three parts, with each addressing key components of a well-balanced evening routine every night and year-round:

- **Part 1: Bedtime Mantras for Relaxation**, the mantras and rituals in the first part of the year, are for relaxation—to give your body and mind a break from the everyday demands of life. This section is designed to support you in taking moments to recalibrate, optimize your energy, rebalance, and tap into calm, so you may more easily fall asleep and stay asleep all night long.

- **Part 2: Bedtime Mantras for Releasing Stress** and the second part of the year features mantras and rituals to not only help you relieve stress but rest and sleep better. It focuses on restful rituals and practices designed to take you out of fight-or-flight mode and recenter yourself to a place of peace. Stress can get the best of us, especially when we focus on all the overwhelming aspects of our responsibilities. Use this section's mantras and tools to calm your nervous system and improve your quality of sleep, so you wake up refreshed and in a better mood.

- **Part 3: Bedtime Mantras for Enjoying Dreams**, the final part of the year, is about dreaming deeply, in your sleep state and waking life alike, to help you enjoy your dreams and rejuvenate your soul. Dreams are the most untapped area of our lives,

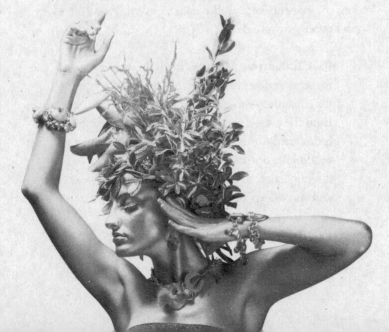

yet their impact is profound: they represent layers of subconscious and conscious awareness, giving insights into deeper meanings of one's mental, physical, emotional, and spiritual well-being. This section celebrates deep sleep by giving you tools to prepare for a good night's rest and make your dreams more potent. It also taps into the layers of a quality life—when you sleep better, you live a more rewarding life. Everything is connected.

BUILDING YOUR
SLEEP-WELLNESS TOOLKIT

I highly recommend creating a designated sleep-wellness toolkit for use with this book and beyond, adding to it as you continue to build your evening wind-down and self-care practice. This list includes some of the items mentioned with the bedtime mantras and their rituals. (Note: an asterisk indicates an item that costs more or may not be readily available. Please work within whatever budget and parameters feel comfortable to you, and as always make it your own by doing what works for you.) Here are some we use in the rituals of this book.

- adaptogens* (relaxing herbs like ashwagandha, reishi, etc.)

- bath oil

- bedding that you enjoy

- bells or bowls* (for sound healing)

- bubble bath (instant awe)

- cacao or cocoa powder

- candles (i.e., tealights or battery powered [safer if you fall asleep!])

- carrier oils* (i.e., almond, coconut, jojoba)

- coloring book (with crayons, colored pencils, etc.)

- color therapy

- crystals and stones* (i.e., amethyst, black tourmaline, lapis, moonstone, pyrite, rose quartz, selenite)

- earplugs

- Epsom salt (for baths)

- essential oils* (i.e., bergamot, jasmine, lavender, lemongrass, palo santo, peppermint, sweet orange, valerian root)

- essential oil diffuser*

- face mask (from the store or homemade [with aloe vera gel and powdered clay*])

- furry friend, your favorite stuffed animal or pet

- healthier bedtime snacks (i.e., cheese and crackers, dark chocolate, fruit, oatmeal, protein shake)

- herbal tea (no caffeine!)

- Himalayan salt lamp*

- houseplants

- incense (including copal resin*)

- journal (with pens, etc.)

- meditation/music apps (i.e., Calm, Mindful, Mindbloom, Happier, SoundCloud, YouTube)

- mug (your favorite oversized one for coffee and teatime)

- pain-relieving topicals* (i.e., CBD oil, Tiger Balm)

- prayer or mala beads or stones

- puzzles (crossword, sudoku, word finds, etc.)

- rubber duckie* (for bath time)

- sketch pad (with pencils, etc.)

- sleep (eye) mask

- sleep-tracking devices* (i.e., wearables like Fitbit)

- smudge bundle/sticks* (i.e., birch bark, sage)

- spray bottle (for oil-infused water)

- stress ball or modeling clay*

- sunrise alarm clock*

- tuning fork(s)* (for sound healing)

- weighted blanket*

- white-noise machine* (or app)

- worry stone

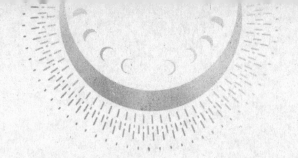

Elevate your self-care practice by taking time out for yourself each evening. Prioritize rest, relaxation, and quality sleep by adding this book to your overall wellness routine—I created it just for you. Journey into more self-love and self-care as you welcome in a more peaceful, calm, well-rested, and healthy version of yourself. You deserve it.

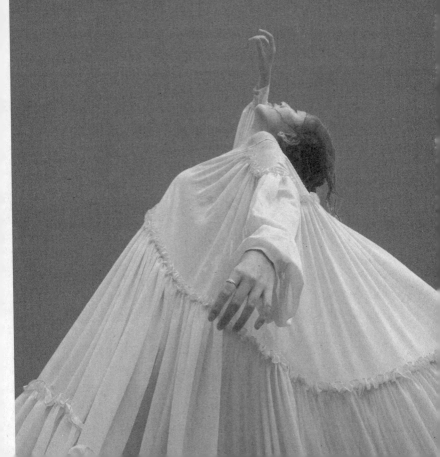

1

BEDTIME MANTRAS FOR RELAXATION

I AM READY TO REST.
ALL IS WELL.

Reflect upon your day and seek comfort in knowing that you have done enough in service to it. Take a deep breath in and surrender to a wave of relaxation, feeling it wash over you. As you breathe out, release any leftover stress or fear-based thoughts carried over from the day. Fall deeper into the evening as you cultivate comfort—you can train your mind to be more at peace with thoughtful intentions and wellness rituals. *Start tonight.*

I calm my mind and balance my heart.
I observe my space, and I am present in the
moment. I relax my mind to drop deeper
into a relaxed state.

RELAXATION RITUAL

Close your eyes and breathe in. Observe your breath to undo the negative effects of a day of multitasking and focus on the present moment. Breathe in loving energy, breathe out worry and fear. Repeat as needed, until you feel grounded and safe.

I FEEL RELAXED AND CONTENT.

Set the intention to "call in" the energy of calm. Watch out for negative thoughts and actively ignore them when they try to reach you. Imagine for a moment that these thoughts are like a negative friend trying to call you: when the phone rings, you don't have to pick up and engage in drama or gossip. Just hit ignore and send this negativity straight to voicemail—through your mind and into the delete folder. For the happy, uplifting friends (thoughts), be available for them. Choose your thoughts the same way you choose your friends.

I am selective with my thoughts, choosing quality over quantity. I choose positive thoughts that support me, and I am only available for those that are kind and loving.

RELAXATION RITUAL

Swap out digital distractions with a meditation. If you find yourself on your digital device, aimlessly browsing the web before bed, tune in to a meditation through a free app (or CD), then turn off all notifications and put your device into "do not disturb" mode. Refocus your energy to the meditation.

I AM THE ONLY ONE RESPONSIBLE FOR MY OWN SENSE OF CALM.

The more we force ourselves to reach a Zen state of mind like the Buddha, the harder it is to reach nirvana; our focus is based on how hard it is to clear our minds of racing thoughts rather than allowing them. Instead of trying to escape these thoughts, consider diving straight into them. Why not face what you've been resisting? (Hint: this is a metaphor for all areas of your life.) That is the true power and purpose of mindfulness—to be so present and aware of the moment that you don't judge anything, especially yourself or your thoughts, nor do you run. Try it tonight.

I sit in stillness and observe what is coming up. I watch these thoughts come and go, attaching to nothing and letting it all be. I am responsible for my own mental state.

RELAXATION RITUAL

Close your eyes and practice nonjudgment as you observe your thoughts, letting them come and go as they are.

I FLOW INSTEAD OF FORCE.

Your life is a series of unfolding events and experiences that shape who you are. When you force outcomes, life feels a lot more burdensome, making you exhausted at times. This impacts your day and evening routines, affecting your ability to fall asleep at night. Look at your life on a timeline, thinking about past pivotal moments, major life events, and the wonderful highlights so far. Watch your life like a movie, allowing yourself to witness the hard times versus reliving them. As you watch your movie, recognize that you've always been able to make it through by tapping into your inner strength and trusting the process.

I relax into my being. I am in flow with the natural rhythm of life and aware that all is in divine, right order.

RELAXATION RITUAL

Tuck yourself into bed and use a weighted blanket (or multiple blankets) to evoke a sense of warmth and calm. As you drift off to sleep, watch and enjoy the highlights of your life movie with curiosity in your mind's eye.

Consistency supports my happiness and health.

You've heard it before: "an apple a day keeps the doctor away." While many of us focus on biting into that delicious, crisp apple, others recognize the importance of eating a wholesome, healthy diet (after all, who doesn't appreciate fewer doctor visits?). The key to this wildly shared message, however, is the power of routine. A healthy lifestyle is all about consistency and regular habits that include the consumption of nutritious foods, engaging in regular physical activity, and getting quality sleep. Research even proves that those with a consistent bedtime routine not only experience improved sleep but improved social skills, academic success, and resilience during times of crisis.[26] So, be proud of yourself! The steps you take tonight are helping support all your tomorrows.

I commit to being better in my bedtime practice, focusing on a quality routine that nourishes my health, inside and out.

Relaxation Ritual

Drink a warm cup of herbal tea before bed and give thanks to yourself for all the ways you've shown up for your body's well-being today.

QUALITY CONNECTIONS ARE AVAILABLE TO ME.

Sometimes we get so caught up in our busy lives that we forget to check in with loved ones. Maintaining quality connections and creating time for meaningful conversations is part of healthy relationships and personal well-being, but when you are stressed out and behind on self-care, it can be especially difficult to prioritize. If it has been a while since you've connected with loved ones, friends, and family, set the intention to touch base with them soon. But make sure you are taking enough time for yourself *first*—that you are not giving too much to others and that they are showing up for you. All relationships require a balance of equal give and take.

*I fall asleep tonight knowing that I prioritize
quality connections and relationships.
I support others and they support me.*

RELAXATION RITUAL

Connect with a loved one over dinner or evening tea, either in person or over the phone. Share a meaningful experience you've had recently and ask about the same from them.

I DO NOT OVERCOMMIT MY TIME. I ALLOW MYSELF TO SLOW DOWN.

Have you overcommitted yourself, saying yes when you wish you would have said no? Many of us overcommit, sometimes because of poor time management and other times because last-minute things come up (the kids need help, the cat gets sick, your car breaks down, etc.). Changing plans or not being able to follow through on your word happens, but if your friends and family have come to expect this, it's time to make some improvements. If you find yourself canceling plans instead of keeping them, start by saying, "Thanks for asking me. Let me get back to you." This way, you make realistic decisions and keep your promises to yourself and others. Commit to moving from "flaky" to "trustworthy" again.

I take my word seriously and honor my commitments. I'm in integrity with myself and others, keeping my promises to both.

RELAXATION RITUAL

Pull out your journal and reflect on a promise you've made yourself and followed through on. How did keeping your word to yourself impact your life?

I DESERVE DEEP, PEACEFUL SLEEP.

Your need for sleep is more than just giving your body rest; it's also a gift to your overthinking mind. When you sleep at night, your ego mind rests and your unconscious mind activates. The unconscious part of your mind is where your memory and automatic skills are held, like the ability to ride a bike: once you learn, you don't really forget—the same way typists or pianists don't have to look at the keys, as the keystrokes have become automatic to them. Learned skills become automatic functions, and just like any skill at which you become proficient, you can train yourself to be a quality sleeper with practice and care.

I relax my mind by establishing a healthy bedtime routine. Each moment of rest is a new opportunity to relax deeper into the night and experience quality sleep.

RELAXATION RITUAL

Play lo-fi music during your evening wind-down routine. Lo-fi music is laid-back, with slow tempos and a relaxed, chilled-out vibe.

THERE IS STRENGTH IN EXPRESSING HOW I FEEL.

If you were denied your emotional experiences growing up, or a positive or negative attribute was put onto feelings (such as "we don't get mad in this house" or "you have nothing to be sad about"), you learned that showing your feelings led to invalidating and painful situations, and likely now avoid their expression altogether. Unfortunately, suppressed emotions get stuffed into your body and never go away. And if you keep suppressing them into adulthood, they can turn into psychological and physical symptoms. If you avoid talking about your feelings or feel distressed when someone asks how you feel, emotional repression could be harming your health and relationships. Reconnect with yourself by exploring your feelings, and trust that you are safe to do so.

My emotions are important indicators of my inner landscape. Feeling my emotions is part of my healing journey and normal human experience.

RELAXATION RITUAL
Practice naming and sharing your emotions with your partner, a family member, or a close friend. Use "I" statements, such as "I feel . . ." and encourage them to share their feelings too.

When I take deep, conscious breaths, my body relaxes.

Breathing is life sustaining yet largely unconscious—an automatic function. Likewise, doing simple breathing techniques throughout the day and evening (a conscious effort) improves your stress response and calms anxiety. Whenever you feel overwhelmed and stressed, use your breath as a tool to come back to your center.

Breathing brings oxygen into your cells, regulating and supporting your body. Naturally, physical and emotional stressors affect how you breathe. Taking moments to consciously focus on your breath calms your central nervous system and sustains you throughout the day.

I take deep, conscious breaths, filling my entire body with oxygen. I feel safe in my body and trust the flow of life. My body relaxes as I breathe in and out.

Relaxation Ritual

Practice box breathing: Breathe in through your nose as you slowly count to four in your head, filling your diaphragm and lungs. Hold your breath for a count of four. Exhale for another count of four. Wait to inhale again for a count of four. Repeat three or four times, feeling yourself relax further with each round.

Setting boundaries is healthy for my well-being.

Having healthy boundaries is the key to healthy relationships; without them, relationships crumble. Holding in opinions and emotions leads to feeling cut off from others, and oversharing feelings leads to codependence and disappointment—not ideal! When you maintain healthy boundaries, you demonstrate self-respect, and this energetically shows others respect.

Boundaries are not intended to keep people out; they are designed to invite people to know where you stand, and it is a vulnerable way to invite people in. Establish clear boundaries with your time, energy, and others to allow yourself to meet your own needs, without giving away your autonomy. A mutual respect for boundaries fosters balanced, thriving connections.

I draw on my own power to activate loving awareness for my time and energy. I do this effortlessly when I have healthy boundaries and share them confidently with those I care about.

Relaxation Ritual

Identify someone in your life with whom you need to set a clear boundary. Set an intention to do so tomorrow, even if it's one small step at a time.

I AM NOT ALONE—I AM CARED FOR, LOVED, AND SUPPORTED.

It may feel easier to do things on your own versus relying on others for help—maybe because you look or feel vulnerable, you are used to being the giver, or you have difficulty trusting others. Whatever the reason, not asking for help can hold you back. Learning how to ask for and receive support is one of the greatest gifts you can give yourself; just make sure you are surrounded by people who consider your best interests. Those who genuinely care want to support you and will do so without making you feel like a burden.

I value my time and my energy, protecting and nurturing both daily. I pay attention to my connections and surround myself with uplifting, supportive, kind people.

RELAXATION RITUAL

Put your pointer fingers to your temples, close your eyes, and ask for your angel guides (whoever you feel aligned with), higher self, higher power, the Universe, God, or your ancestors to come through and share any message or wisdom they have for you at this time. Be willing to receive what they deliver.

My day went well, and I feel settled.

Reflect on the day by celebrating everything that went well, making a mental list or even writing it down. Now bring your attention to the present moment, letting the evening bring you into a deeper sense of gratitude as it comes to a close. If today didn't go the way you'd hoped, recognize that tomorrow is a new day full of new opportunities to do things differently. Release the past day, and let it be done. Turn your attention to your breath and invite calm energy to wash over you.

I sit content in this moment. I allow myself to relax and leave behind the tension of the day. I am no longer in the past. I am here—now— and I feel satisfied.

Relaxation Ritual

Take a warm bath or shower before bed. As you finish, consciously focus on releasing the day as the water spirals down the drain. Focus on gratitude as you settle deeper into the night.

I AM GRATEFUL FOR MY HEALTH.

Celebrate the aspects of your well-being that feel alive, vibrant, and well. One of the most overlooked aspects is quality sleep, and your rest routine requires a healthy approach for you to feel happy. When you rest well at night, your body relaxes, reducing the burdens of physical and emotional pain. Parts of your body may not be in optimal alignment, but this doesn't mean you have to focus on them solely; focusing on physical pain or whatever isn't going well only amplifies the struggle. No matter where you are in your health journey, take time each day and night to appreciate your life as a gift.

I appreciate my quality sleep and prioritize it—it is a pillar of optimal wellness and health. I make each night a relaxing experience of gratitude for my body and my ultimate well-being.

RELAXATION RITUAL

In your journal, write down five things you are grateful for in your health and physical body, such as "I am grateful for my strong legs," etc.

WITH EACH PASSING BREATH, I AM MORE AT EASE.

It's impossible to relax in a chronic stress-response mode. You could be burdened by the demands of the world, work expectations, past trauma, or personal worries, all of which keep you from accessing inner peace. When out of balance, you may experience elevated cortisol levels, which make it extra hard to relax and fall asleep. Take a moment to use your breath to return to center: breathe in calm, exhale stress; breathe in calm, exhale stress. Do this as often as you need to become more centered in the here and now.

I destress and decompress, doing more with less effort. I stay calm in all situations and let my breath bring me back into balance. Calm is my main intention.

RELAXATION RITUAL

Lying in bed, stretch out your legs, flex your ankles, and rotate your feet. Lift your legs up and down together, bending at the hips, and then bend at your knees, bringing them toward your chest and away again. Thank your feet and legs for carrying you through another day.

I TAKE THE TIME
I NEED TO HEAL.

There is no expiration date on healing the heart and mending what has been lost or broken. Whether you're healing physically, emotionally, or mentally, it takes time—as you heal, you grow and expand. If your mind or body is out of alignment, your health will decline. If you are not taking time to rest both the body and the mind, the healing process may feel forced or hindered. When you rest, you give yourself time to integrate the changes you are activating.

Healing is my priority—I am connected to this journey and the evolution of my expansive self. I do not force or try to make anything fit. In this moment, all is as it should be, for all is right when I tend to my body, mind, and soul.

RELAXATION RITUAL

Go to your bookshelf and pick a book you feel called to. Open a page—any page you feel guided to—and read a sentence or two. This is a message the universe has for you.

I SLEEP WITH THE RHYTHM OF NATURE.

Be honest: how many hours of screen time did you have last week? (*Gulp!*) Screen-time statistics show us where we can improve. If stress has been getting the best of you, consider ditching digital devices for a few hours this week, saying *sayonara* to screen time and hello to more *green* time. In less than five minutes, you can start to feel better. According to research, nature boosts your mood fast, reducing stress, improving mental health, and inducing quality sleep.[27] When you connect with nature, you align to the natural order of all things. Let nature be your natural stress reliever and ritual for better rest.

Nature heals me. Like the wind blowing through the air, I am not attached to anything. It shows me how to be free of worry and uncertainty.

RELAXATION RITUAL

Do some couch cuddle time with a loved one (partner, child, or furry friend) and a nature-inspired bedtime story. Take turns sharing a favorite memory in nature. (If you prefer, you can do this same ritual with yourself and your journal.)

EVERYTHING IS IN PERFECT ORDER.

When is the last time you worried about something over which you had no control? To release yourself from the mental prison of overthinking, worry, and uncertainty, focus your mind on what is going well in your life. Life feels a lot better when you pay attention to the quality of your thoughts. If possible, clear your schedule tonight, allowing yourself to relax in the wonder of all that is well. The Universe is always in perfect order, especially when you listen to yourself and trust your own judgment. Rest is possible when you let go of worry. Tonight, recognize all is perfection just as it is.

I see clearly through the illusions of pain and past all worry. The clouds of judgment, fear, and uncertainty dissipate. As I relax fully into the moment, I know I am supremely guided.

RELAXATION RITUAL

Expel and calm any excess energy or fidgeting by squeezing a stress ball or molding a ball of clay, Silly Putty, or Play-Doh with your hands.

In mind and body, I am strong.

You are far more powerful than you know—you have immense strength within and around you. Give yourself permission to feel this power, and trust that you can overcome anything in life, especially when you prioritize the force and connection to your own mind and body. Take time each night to focus on your mind and body and how strong you are—on how much you have already endured in this life. This strength is your personal source of inspiration, honor, and trust.

I listen to my body's wisdom and my mind's wise guidance—they always know what is best for me. I honor their innate gifts by giving them quality rest at night.

RELAXATION RITUAL

Close your eyes, and relax your forehead and jaw. Imagine yourself as a superhero. What cause do you fight for, and what is your superpower? Honor this strength through a related activity this week (like helping others in need, such as donating to or volunteering for a charity that resonates with you).

I LET GO OF THE DAY.

Reflect upon your day and observe how your experiences unfolded. Do you feel things could have gone better? Are you ruminating on something you didn't say or wish you had said differently? Allow your mind to acknowledge these things, then return to the now—the present. Your mind wants to fix, judge, analyze, but your soul wants to relax, accept, and release. Let go of the day by focusing on what is right rather than what is wrong. Trust that the stressful situations turned out fine and all will be better tomorrow.

I let go of the day and anything that stood in my way. I free myself from the pain of the past and learn from its lessons. I am connected to the now, free of stress, worry, and concern about anything or anyone.

RELAXATION RITUAL

Create a let-go playlist of music that inspires you. As you listen, write in your journal a list of all the things, people, places, fears, etc. that you are ready to release.

I EXPRESS AND ADDRESS THE NEEDS OF MY INNER CHILD.

As adults, we have to relearn how to be there for our wounded inner child—the part of us that didn't feel seen, loved, or acknowledged in childhood. This looks and feels like reclaiming lost parts of yourself, giving yourself permission to play, cry, explore, hide, be curious, and more. The version of you that has been afraid to express your needs and share them honestly with others requires *your* attention and love first. There is no need to hide from your range of emotions anymore; you are free to dive into them fully. Give yourself permission to be who you are, starting *now*—tonight. Reach out to that inner child and hold them close tonight, safe and sound at last.

I am in touch with my inner child and nurture their needs. I do not abandon or ignore any part of myself.

RELAXATION RITUAL

Before bed, grab a pen and your journal, and connect with your inner child by writing or drawing a picture of a heartfelt message to your younger self.

I CONTRACT MY ENERGY BEFORE REACTING. I ONLY RESPOND WITH LOVE.

Are you proud of how you showed up in the world today? Was there a situation where you wish you had responded with more compassion and kindness? Tonight is an opportunity for you to look at the energy exchanges in your life and refrain from attacking, blaming, or shaming others. When someone says something to you about your character, you may want to defend yourself; realize, however, that what other people say is more about them—it rarely has anything to do with you. Respond when you feel love pulsing through your body, seeking connection over control.

When people tell me things about myself, I don't take on this truth. I use this opportunity to understand where they are coming from and get closer to them. I choose to respond in love.

RELAXATION RITUAL

Choose a person in your life with whom you have been in conflict. Try to send them love and pray for their well-being. Imagine they are sending this good energy back to you.

I AM SELF-LOYAL—I DO NOT BETRAY MYSELF TO CONNECT WITH OTHERS.

Are you being honest with others about who you really are, or are you hiding aspects of yourself, worried they won't accept you as you are? Instead of needing others to love you in the way that you show up for them, turn that love back to you. If others are not there for you, it could be because you have abandoned aspects of your own nature in exchange for their approval. What you want is connection, meaning, and honesty in your relationships, but you must first give these things to yourself. Make a promise that you will never betray or abandon yourself—that your loyalty is always to you, first and foremost.

I show up as my authentic self and let others see the real me. I choose to acknowledge and embrace all of me, exactly as I am.

RELAXATION RITUAL

Light a candle—a symbol of your special light in the world—and consciously focus on what you appreciate about your individuality and what makes you unique.

I CHOOSE TO EXPLORE MY FEELINGS—THERE ARE LESSONS TO BE LEARNED.

When you move into your evening routine, you want to be free of mental stress, but life doesn't make it easy to do this. If you're overwhelmed with chronic overthinking, it could be because an emotion wants to be felt. When we avoid our feelings, our minds can run wild with ruminations as a distraction. Feel your emotions in your body by allowing yourself to let go, drop your shoulders, breathe in deeply, and cry. Tears are an important part of healing any pain.

I let the anxiety of my mind subside by dropping consciously into my body and feeling what needs to be felt. I trust the process and know it is safe. When I feel, I heal.

RELAXATION RITUAL

Fix your mind on a loss in your life—whatever shows up. Allow yourself to cry and release stagnant energy. It is important to grieve—change and loss are a part of life. And this physical release of sadness is healing in itself.

I SEND HEALING THOUGHTS AND ENERGY TO A LOVED ONE IN NEED.

Who needs extra love and care right now? This could be someone you know personally or someone you have never met before, even from the public arena (a famous person, actor, or politician). Sending love and prayers to others is a powerful way to join together and offer support. Devoting your thoughts to someone in need is a beautiful method for healing too. Help yourself and others by caring for them with your actions, thoughts, and intentions. As you send them love, you increase your own vibration and open a channel for the same love to come back to you.

I support others with love. I am connected to my heart and use my energy for good. I uplift others by first uplifting myself.

RELAXATION RITUAL

Send positive energy and prayers to someone who is important to you (a friend, partner, family member, coworker, mentor), dedicating tonight's self-love practice to them. As you send uplifting energy their way, you, too, will be uplifted.

I RELEASE STAGNANT ENERGY AND LET REST WASH OVER ME.

Your body is like an antenna, attracting whatever it is vibrationally aligned to. When you focus on raising your vibration with good thoughts, healthy eating, quality sleep, and a community of growth-focused, supportive people, you attract healthier opportunities and people to you. Conversely, when your vibration is lowered by negative thoughts, eating processed food, and a community of energy vampires, you will naturally feel more drained. Your health and wellness are impacted by the frequency to which you tune your vessel, impacting your need for rest and energy accordingly.

I rid myself of low vibrations and negative thoughts, and align to what serves my highest good. I release my body of energetic heaviness and let good-feeling vibrations purify me.

RELAXATION RITUAL

Tonight, consider the feng shui of your bedroom. It may be too late in the evening to actually move the room's contents, but you can still take a moment to examine how to rearrange things for better energetic flow in the future.

I AM OKAY WITH NOT BEING OKAY.

If you're going through a lot right now, your mind, body, and soul need a break. It's okay to not be okay. Sit for a moment in the energy of feeling "off." Give yourself permission to fully experience the feeling of *not okay*. When a loved one asks you how you are, instead of brushing them off, tell them the truth—you are feeling down, overwhelmed, afraid. Let your inner circle see how you really are. This is different than dumping your struggles on them; it is about not isolating yourself in sadness anymore. Sometimes being honest with ourselves means admitting that we are not okay.

My emotions are important indicators of where I am imbalanced—of what needs more attention and care. I lean on others by being honest and accept myself as I am.

RELAXATION RITUAL

Before bed, grab a worry stone and hold it under tap water for a few minutes to cleanse it. Put it under your pillow to welcome more positive vibrations and support as you rest.

I RECOGNIZE MY TRIGGERS AND GIVE MYSELF GRACE.

Mentally strong people know how to combat negative thoughts with positive, uplifting ones, and physically strong people know how to listen to the body to provide what it needs (exercise, good food, sleep, etc.). But when our emotional side experiences pain, the next steps get clouded. Being emotional is often considered weakness, so we "power through," stuffing the pain inside until it has nowhere else to go. Is it any wonder why we get maxed out and reactive?

Work through triggers by taking inspiration from mentally and physically strong people: acknowledge your emotions and exercise their healthy expression. Be compassionate and patient with yourself—emotional healing takes time. Trust in the strength of grace.

My ability to see things clearly is my strength. I honor my emotional landscape with more love, joy, and ease.

RELAXATION RITUAL

Sit cross-legged on the floor or on the edge of your bed. Place your hands on your knees with your palms facing up, with a spirit of openness. Acknowledge your emotions and see them as a source of strength as you release them from your body.

Even when my emotions are heightened, I am safe.

Your emotions are very powerful indicators intended to guide you back to safety. Tune in to them to help you navigate life, especially in times of uncertainty. If you feel anxious, worried, concerned, or fearful, feel these emotions fully, allowing them to lead you toward a greater understanding of your truth and surrounding situations. We are often taught to avoid our emotions and emotional pain, but your feelings are part of your body's calibration system. Connect with the emotions that come up throughout the day and process them each night. As you do this, you will experience more balance, wisdom, and peace.

I welcome my emotions as I process them. I feel them fully to get the valuable information they have to offer. I listen closely to my inner knowingness and trust its guidance.

Relaxation Ritual

Do something tonight to consciously create your sleep setting. Choose the color of your bedding, sheet set, or the clothing you wear to bed—anything that helps you feel calm, protected, and secure.

I TAKE CARE OF MYSELF BY PRIORITIZING MY SLEEP.

When you show up for yourself throughout the day, you rest more fully at night. As one of the most important yet overlooked aspects of your health routine, it is essential that you focus on getting enough quality sleep nightly. You will know you've had quality rest when you sleep close to eight hours, don't wake up often, and feel well rested when you wake up in the morning. Make sleep part of your self-care routine tonight—there's no good reason to wait!—and bask in the beautiful energy of a well-rested you.

When I need to rest, I surrender to my bed and create a supportive sleep routine. I wake up refreshed and confident because I prioritize my needs and I take care of me.

RELAXATION RITUAL

Set the intention to prioritize your sleep starting tonight! With an app or in your journal, track your sleep schedule for the next week, including your observations of how you feel as a result. Reflect on the patterns and make any adjustments.

LOVE IS MY LEADER, GUIDING ME THROUGH EACH DAY AND NIGHT.

You have loving awareness all around you in the form of energy, extending out in your auric field. This energy uplifts you and can support those around you, but right now, it is time to focus on yourself. Let love lead you into your nightly routine, caring for you and your body with nurturing activities that invite you to wind down with ease. As you surround yourself with loving energy, you are protected from negative thoughts and low-vibrational situations. Let love be your guide throughout the day and into the night.

Love is my embodied awareness.
I tune out negativity and turn up positivity.
I am love in action.

RELAXATION RITUAL

Starting with your fingertips on one side of your body, send love to all your body parts (inside and out) as you travel up to your head and then down to your fingertips on the other side. Imagine every one of your cells embodied with this loving energy and peace.

I AM SECURE AND AT PEACE.

To be secure in a chaotic world requires a steadfast connection to your inner self and your faith. Who you really are is not what you do or how people see you; it is your essence—your unique spirit—and your character. When you tap into your true self and allow this to lead you forward, your safety comes into perfect alignment with the peace that lives within. You are always secure when you put your trust in yourself and the universe. As you go to bed tonight, relax into your body and become aware of the reliable rhythm and warmth of your heart.

I am secure within myself. I rest in my body with peace as my personal power. I do not need the outside world to give me what I already have within. I am secure as I am.

RELAXATION RITUAL

Invite peace and stillness as you settle into bed. Find and listen to a binaural-beat playlist to calm your body and mind.

TRUST AND PEACE ARE WITHIN ME.

It isn't always possible to trust other people, and you will find yourself in situations where you are on guard. Reflect upon your day and consider how and where you felt uneasy or wronged. Did someone do something that felt unjust or unfair? Did you do something unjust or unfair to someone else? Look within yourself to see if and how you are betraying or not trusting yourself; what you experience day to day is often a manifestation of your own thoughts, projections, and inner knowing. Trust yourself above all, knowing that peace must first come from within.

I prioritize trust in my relationship with myself, and as I do, I build stronger, healthier, more peaceful connections with others.

RELAXATION RITUAL

Tonight, put a few drops of your favorite essential oil on a washcloth with warm water and put it on your face for a few minutes while you lay in bed. (Using an oil diffuser by your bed is another option.)

BETTER SLEEP MEANS BETTER SUCCESS, HARMONY, AND WELLNESS.

Getting sleep is more than just resting your body and mind; it is an avenue to success and harmony in your life. Imagine how good you feel when you're well rested. Getting a great night's sleep affects every point of the day that follows. If you're working toward a specific goal in life, looking for an outcome that will bring greater success and abundance, start to recognize how your sleep plays into this manifestation. Sleep peacefully for a solid eight hours every night, and your entire life will feel more grounded and focused. Even better, you will see your achievements manifest easier.

My rest is my sanctuary, and my sleep is my success. I achieve proper rest at night; I achieve greatness in life.

RELAXATION RITUAL

Get creative with your sleep routine by creating a game of it tonight. Set up the "rules" for quality sleep and your ultimate goal, then track your success, giving yourself a prize when you achieve your goal.

I AM FREE OF FEAR.

When clouded by fear, we are trapped in illusion—a distraction from our true state of inner peace—adding to our mental angst and pain. Look at your own life and see if you are grasping, manipulating, forcing, or trying to make things fit. Are you giving away your power to life circumstances, operating from a passive hope of receiving versus being an active participant in taking inspired action toward your heart's desires? If so, you may be stuck in fear and operating from a place of lack. When and if this happens, take note and align to the joyful promise of your life with pure delight in your heart. This act in itself can free you from the fear that's holding you back.

I am the light, love, and promise in my life.
I am inspiration and truth, and I am strong.

RELAXATION RITUAL

As you fall asleep, create a bedtime story in your head about being your own hero, living fearless and without bounds in your waking life.

My needs are important. I honor them daily.

Honoring your needs means setting and honoring boundaries with others at work, at home, in your social life, and elsewhere, so you can take better care of yourself. Are you drinking enough water, eating a wholesome diet, getting daily movement, and practicing self-love and self-compassion? Are you spending enough time focusing on your hobbies and personal growth? Sometimes we feel exhausted simply because we aren't showing up for ourselves in all the ways necessary to keep up with our daily lives. Tonight, focus on taking care of your needs and prioritizing *you*. You are worth it and you deserve it.

I listen to my inner guide daily. I recognize my needs and their effect on my overall well-being. I honor them and myself.

Relaxation Ritual

As a method of self-care, drink a glass of water before bed and bless the water as you slowly sip it. Feel it nourishing your body and your whole being, including all your cells and your soul.

I AM A PORTAL FOR DIVINE INSPIRATION.

Becoming who you are requires nothing more than surrendering to what is. Your unique essence is already within; you simply lose touch with it at times. When you feel powerless, tap into the innate inspiration of your soul. You are a portal to the divine Source, and you have access to its inspiration at any time. Remember your personal power. Take a moment to relax into the present, and connect with the peace that comes from living in harmony with your true self. Let this vibration lead you into peaceful days and restful nights.

I breathe in all the goodness available to me—it flows through each cell to achieve the highest alignment and ultimate collaboration. I am the peace and light I seek in the world.

RELAXATION RITUAL

Before bed tonight, grab some crayons or colored pencils and color in a coloring book. Let your creative inspiration shine in a spirit of play with the world and all that exists.

I REST SAFELY IN MY BODY, TRUSTING ALL IS WELL.

Next time you feel triggered, take a moment to be aware of where you feel unsafe in your body. What is your mind saying about your current situation? You may know that you are in no real harm, but in times of distress, your body reacts by going into overprotective mode. Healing takes time, but when you reconnect your anxious mind to your triggered body, you start to affirm that all is okay in this moment. Use your breath to connect to the here and now. Pay attention to your body's clues, and trust yourself and your breath fully.

*I am safe in my body, and I find peace within.
I recognize my triggers as opportunities to
heal, and I trust myself fully.*

RELAXATION RITUAL

Balance yourself before bed. Sit in a comfortable position, close your eyes, and imagine a gentle stream of emerald-green light flowing up from the base of your spine and out of the top of your head. Gently chant *om* until you feel grounded and safe.

I FIND SOLACE BY RELAXING MY MIND.

Have you ever watched a cat or a dog just sit and stare at nothing in particular? They appear calm, cool, and totally collected—without a care in the world. You, too, can be cool as a cucumber when you remove yourself from the constant influence of external stimuli and stress. We spend so much time staring at screens and processing incoming information that we forget to protect ourselves from technology and information overload. When you rest, you reset. Your brain relaxes as your body restores. Give both the opportunity for quality sleep tonight.

I rest my body and my mind daily. I relax deeper into the evening by relaxing deeper into myself. Deep peace lives in my solace and slumber.

RELAXATION RITUAL

Tonight, turn off or silence all digital devices a few hours before bedtime, putting them out of reach. Let your mind wind down with something simple, like reading a book in a comfy chair, and your body will soon follow.

After all I've been through, I deserve rest.

You are doing so much to be there for others while showing up the best you can for yourself—and often, it may feel like it's never enough. Tonight is a reminder that you do not need to work so hard to be seen, understood, and loved; you are already loved as you are, and you deserve to embody this, which you can when you rest. If you find yourself in a situation where things did not go as planned, view the closing out of this past cycle as a healing process—one that requires rest before you can enter a new phase of your life. Be patient and trust the process.

Tranquility is mine when I allow things to be as they are in the present moment. I release the past and the future. I honor myself and the needs of my overall well-being.

Relaxation Ritual

Use your bedding to wrap yourself up like a caterpillar nestling into its cocoon. As you drift off to sleep, imagine yourself waking as a beautiful butterfly, fully transformed and healed.

I AM WHO I AM, AND MY PATH IS PERFECT FOR ME.

If you've ever felt resentful because your coworker got the promotion that you were hoping for or your sister got married first, you are selling yourself short. Relationships can quickly unravel at the hand of the green-eyed monster—jealousy. Remember that we all have our own life path—one that is for our highest good. Sometimes we don't get what we want simply because it doesn't align to our timeline. Every choice you make has the option to take a turn onto the path of fear, greed, jealousy, and competition or a turn onto the path of light, love, peace, harmony, and cooperation. Align your choices to your values, and watch your life transform.

I love myself wholly and am grateful for my life's unique path. I am exactly where I am supposed to be.

RELAXATION RITUAL

As you relax into bed and close your eyes for a good night's sleep, wrap yourself in gratitude for your life's blessings. Focus on feeling secure in your body and on your path by feeling the love in your heart.

It's safe for me to be my authentic self.

When you share your thoughts and feelings with others freely and sincerely, with no agenda or expectations, you offer the gift of your true, authentic self. Even if others don't understand you and respond in kind, it doesn't mean you are not amazing—your worth is not dependent on others seeing or knowing your value. It's your role to show others your own self-respect and self-worth, especially in the face of discord and adversity. Be your true self no matter what, embracing yourself regardless of others' opinions or approval. Shine your light boldly and brightly, without fear or shame.

Authenticity fuels the light of my soul and shines brightly through my actions, feelings, and thoughts. I show up with love and feel safe to share my true self.

Relaxation Ritual

Mist your pillow with a lavender essential oil spray before going to bed. Fluff your pillow and breathe in calm, releasing the day's burdens with every exhale as you reflect on how you showed up for yourself today with self-love, respect, and worth.

I LET IT BREATHE. I LET IT LEAVE.

The day is over—you are done. Check it off the list—it is complete. If there is anything you are holding on to, it is time to let it go. The real reason you're grasping and energetically attaching yourself to something that has expired is because you are still in the past version of you. Instead of blocking yourself from new opportunities, trust the release, then let go. Let it breathe. Let it leave. Your life is happening in the now, not then. Once you detach from the situation, you begin to heal; and in your healing, you reveal the lesson that needed to be learned. Free yourself from the energetic tangle of unmet expectations by opening yourself to new growth and a better tomorrow.

I let go of anything that is not mine to carry.
I leave the past in the past and free myself
for new opportunities.

RELAXATION RITUAL

Smudge your bedroom with palo santo or sage to purify the air, releasing your space of old, dense energy.

I OPTIMIZE MY SLEEP.
MY SLEEP IS MY SANCTUARY.

How did you sleep last night? Without doubt, disrupted sleep and poor sleep quality negatively impact our quality of life in small and big ways. Understanding sleep health and one's personal sleep patterns can greatly turn this around, however. Major advances in sleep research have identified tangible steps we can take nightly to improve our sleep experience. Investing in the emerging sleep-sensing technologies like wearables and airables (wireless tech) can enhance a mindful nightly routine. Merge science and spirituality to optimize your sleep and find the happy medium that works best for you.

I harness the power of science and mindfulness to create a sleep routine that is suitable for me. My sleep is my nightly sanctuary.

RELAXATION RITUAL

Make optimal sleep your focus tonight by doing some research on new sleep technologies to see what might be available to you within your budget and preferences. Before going to bed, always remember the power of your breath as you breathe in thanks and love for this sleep sanctuary you maintain.

46

I CHOOSE TO BE FREE OF DRAMA.

It can be impossible to maintain a sense of tranquility when the people around you are drowning in drama or focused on creating problems rather than solving them. Tonight is an opportunity to look at those with whom you spend most of your time, at home and at work. Do the members of either group stir up trouble, gossip, or cause chaos? Are you able to feel released in their company? Is your circle chill like a day at the beach or like a blizzard in the arctic? Start to pay more attention to how you feel around certain people, and use discernment with your interactions. Are you energized or drained after you spend time with them? It doesn't take long for the latter to take a toll. Remove yourself from drama and choose calm, restorative connections.

I am the company I keep. I surround myself with supportive people who care for and respect me.

RELAXATION RITUAL

Make gratitude part of your bedtime practice tonight. Write a thank-you note to the most supportive person in your life and send it to them tomorrow.

MY DAY IS DONE, AND I WELCOME TIME WITH MYSELF.

If there is a situation from today that is still on your mind and causing you stress, detach from it by focusing on self-awareness. To be self-aware means you understand your feelings, thoughts, and behaviors and monitor them regularly. You recognize that your actions have an impact on others and that your value is separate from them. Self-awareness is a life skill that allows you to recognize any limitations (thoughts, actions, etc.) that might be holding you back and improve upon them. Take some time to check in with yourself tonight and let go of whatever remains from the day.

I am self-aware and comfortable in my body. The day is done, and I am thankful for this time with myself.

RELAXATION RITUAL

Take a moon bath before bed. Go outside or sit by a window, close your eyes, and imagine the moonlight washing over you, its energetic rays flooding over and recharging you, removing negativity and worries.

I BASK IN THE MOONLIGHT AND EMBRACE THE MORNING SUNLIGHT GLOW.

The body's natural clock and brain chemistry are affected by light neurotransmitters and hormones that impact our overall well-being. Believe it or not, a good night's sleep starts first thing in the morning, when we wake up. Starting your day with natural light helps you feel more productive and balanced throughout the entire day.[28] Take some time tomorrow morning to bask in the morning light and give thanks for all that is well. The phototherapy may be just what you need to sleep better and feel more alert during the day.

I invite the morning light to illuminate my heart and my home. I am a beloved part of the natural world, and it is a beloved part of me.

RELAXATION RITUAL

Give yourself some extra time in the morning by setting out your clothes for tomorrow before bed. Use the time to step outside and recharge in the light of a new day (for five to ten minutes, if possible).

I FEEL ACCOMPLISHED WHEN I LIE DOWN TO SLEEP.

There are certain daily productivity hacks to optimize your workflow, and there is none more tried-and-true than the mighty to-do list. Not only does it feel oh-so satisfying to write things down and then check them off, but moving forward on mini goals throughout the day gives a sense of accountability and accomplishment. One of the psychological benefits of making lists is to clarify and prioritize goals. As you tick off the list, your confidence increases—little self-esteem boosters like this are always welcome! Use this tool whenever you feel scattered or stuck in your head. It even works well when it comes to your sleep health, freeing your mind for rest when the day is done.

I sleep more and worry less. My bedtime routine is the last important to-do on my list.

RELAXATION RITUAL

Tonight, empty your mind for rest by making a to-do list of everything you need to do tomorrow. When it feels complete, commit to setting it aside and being done for the night.

I RELEASE MYSELF FROM SELF-JUDGMENT.

Are you spending time in your head, doubting or criticizing yourself? The energy you spend on harsh self-judgment takes away from your quality of life. When you focus on what you dislike about yourself, you lower your vibration. Negative thoughts have energy and power in them—a direct attack on your physical and mental well-being. Consider a more loving approach by seeing yourself through the lens of love—the way you would a beloved child or pet. Extend unconditional love and compassion to yourself to release the burden of self-inflicted pain and judgment. You deserve this kind of love always—every day and every night.

I release the pain of judgment and shame of my ego to embrace my true essence of love. Love frees me of all pain.

RELAXATION RITUAL

Wrap your evening in a loving exchange. Go to your pet or a loved one (or a mirror), look into their eyes, and say, "I love you." As they gaze back at you, see your reflection in their eyes, free of judgment and full of love.

I BRAVELY FACE MY SHADOWS WITH COMPASSION.

Many of us are making our way through life with a limited awareness of the teaching and lessons that have been passed down to us. If your parents operated from their shadow selves, then they most likely passed on unhealthy, wounded, or toxic traits to you. Tonight is an opportunity to look at your own red flags. Do you hide your feelings, ignore your needs, or put others first, even when you are exhausted and overworked? Or maybe you ignore others or take flight during conflict instead of staying to work it out? Perhaps you thrive off drama and try to manipulate others to get what you want? We all have shadow parts of us that require healing. Pay attention to yours with kindness, self-awareness, and love.

I choose to see my shadows and consciously address them. I am doing the best I can, and I strive to keep evolving.

RELAXATION RITUAL

Lighten your mood tonight by watching one of your favorite funny or feel-good childhood TV shows or movies.

MY BODY IS LIGHT AND LOVED.

Your body is a vessel of energy, and you can only hold so much until you need to rest, release, and restore. As you move through life, you pick up and hold on to energy from others as well as yourself, both of which can get buried in your body, along with unmet expectations and demands—the weight of the past. Unprocessed feelings like shame and blame also get stuck in your body, and this pressure builds up. Fortunately, each night brings the opportunity to release the pressure valve and let the unnecessary energy go. Make this your focus tonight.

My body is a magnet to positive energy and a barrier to negative energy. I love my body and rest it nightly, feeling light and free.

RELAXATION RITUAL

Release the energy from the day before going to bed. Breathe in deeply, then make an O shape with your mouth as you breathe out, like a hose releasing pressure. Do this as often as you need, day or night, to expel unwanted energy.

MY EMOTIONS FLOW THROUGH ME FREELY, WITHOUT JUDGMENT.

Are you someone who learned at a young age to suppress your feelings to keep the peace? If so, it's possible you have become a people pleaser. You may feel an internal sadness that is really masking anger from putting others' needs before your own. It's normal to feel angry when healing begins. Tonight, sit with this anger—it's the fuel to alchemize years of ignoring your own light. The more you stand up for yourself and your needs, the more you realize how much you matter. Let your emotions flow through you freely, without judgment.

My anger is the catalyst toward healing the emotions I have suppressed. I welcome my emotions and release self-judgment and shame.

RELAXATION RITUAL

Tonight, pull out your journal and reflect on how you speak to yourself when you're feeling angry. Is it different than how you express anger with others? Is there anything you'd like to change about this self-talk? Conclude with a statement of self-love, compassion, and kindness.

I INVITE POSITIVE ENERGY TO RECHARGE MY BODY AND MY SPIRIT.

Imagine energy as a highway of awesomeness, and you're cruising down its sunset lane. A flow of divine energy is available to you at all times. As you make your way into the evening, bring this energy into your nightly routine; this essence of ease and carefree joy is at your disposal.

Each feeling has a frequency to it, and you get to choose which feeling you tune in to. What frequency would you like to invite in tonight? Joy? Relaxation? Play? Each night before you sleep, invite positive energy to flow through every pore and touch every cell of your body, until you resonate its essence completely.

My frequency is higher when I choose good-feeling vibrations. I release my burdens with positive flow. All is well when I drop from my head into my heart and embrace myself fully.

RELAXATION RITUAL

Tonight, play a soothing, favorite song and as you listen, focus on its positive energy flooding your body and dancing within every cell.

I TAKE TIME TO ENJOY MY SACRED SPACE.

There is nowhere else you need to be, and there is nothing more for you to do. Right here, right now, is all there is. You may feel rushed to find a quick fix or to move around the uncomfortable aspects of life rather than following the path that goes through this discomfort. Any pain you feel in your life is a disconnection from self. Return to you by taking rest seriously and prioritizing your well-being through relaxation. Relaxing into the evening in your sacred space is the only thing on your to-do list tonight.

*I let go of outside pressures and my need
to do anything else or be anywhere else;
I am at home in my body—I embrace my
current place. I care for myself through
the sacred space of my heart.*

RELAXATION RITUAL

Create a sleep altar close to your bed. You can add stones, feathers, photos, plants—anything that evokes a sense of comfort and relaxation at bedtime.

I HAVE THE COURAGE TO ADMIT MY MISTAKES.

Your feelings are valid and hiding them serves no one, especially when you make a mistake. It takes courage to take accountability. Is there an area of your life where you feel you have made a mistake and are having a hard time moving past it? Ruminating on past experiences keeps you stuck in the past, feeling regret over mistakes that are over and done with. Be honest with yourself about the life lessons gained from this experience—we develop new perspectives through hardships. Have the courage to face your mistakes, then forgive yourself and move on.

I have the strength to admit when I am wrong and own up to my mistakes. I live in truth, not regret, and thrive from the lessons in hardship.

RELAXATION RITUAL

Water your plants to clear your conscience before bed. As you lovingly pour the water into the soil of each plant, forgive yourself for a mistake you've made and are ready to release.

I HAVE BEEN BLESSED ALL ALONG.

There are shifts happening inside of you—your circumstances have changed because of newfound gratitude and love within your heart. You may have found yourself in a conflict that felt uncomfortable, and the uncertainty of life may have brought on new levels of anxiety and stress. But when you focus on gratitude and use the skills you have, you will always make it through. Rise above uncertainty to see that there are blessings around you at all times. Your shifting perspective has been your lifeline all along. Embrace the blessings among the changes, and know that all truly is well.

I am thankful for my life and all that is.
I appreciate each chapter of my life and
value its lessons, no matter what I am going
through. I am blessed beyond belief.

RELAXATION RITUAL

As you fall asleep tonight, try counting sheep in a new manner: each sheep represents a blessing in your life. Count your blessings of soft, warm love.

I AM STRONGER THAN MY FEAR-BASED THOUGHTS.

You are not your thoughts, yet the thoughts of your ego want you to think they are real. When you are anxious, you are worried about the unknown future or thinking about the unwanted outcomes of the past. But you are so much stronger than these illusions! Pay attention to the types of thoughts you have and the ways you're handling—or not handling—them. Are you distracting yourself with unnecessary tasks? Don't run from your anxiety; it is merely an imbalance of energy and thoughts—an opportunity for recalibration. Begin with gratitude for their messages and focus on positive, loving thoughts.

My anxiety is here to show me what I need to release. I am stronger than I realize—the greatest champion of my life! Fear is no match for my love and resilience.

RELAXATION RITUAL

Tonight, in your journal, identify what is making you the most anxious in your life right now. Now make a plan to take action tomorrow—what steps will you take?

ALL CONFLICT IS BEHIND ME.

Difficult, karmic periods of life can be turbulent. Imagine yourself as a ship out at sea—you must learn how to navigate the rough waters to get through to the calm ones. As you learn the lessons with each hardship, however, grace is bestowed upon you; and just like that, you emerge stronger than ever before. This strength has been inside you all along. You've overcome the toughest cycles of your entire life and for this moment, celebrate your strength. Think about a recent rough patch and the life lessons learned as you settle in for the night. Trust that your ship always sails toward calmer waters, inside and out.

I persevere, I made it through, I am stronger and more steady than ever. I feel the internal shift as I rise up into more love. I navigate forward with clarity and confidence. I am powerful and wiser than ever before.

RELAXATION RITUAL

Untether yourself energetically before bed. Identify a person you've been in recent conflict with and imagine a white crystal thread connecting you. Send them forgiveness and cut the thread, leaving the karmic connection behind.

My mind is at rest, my body is at ease.

The state of our mental health and our activity on social media is connected, and it's possible that the anxiety you've experienced lately is tied to your digital habits. When scrolling through your feeds, you may feel a sense of community in all the updates, highlights, and shared posts, yet it often generates the opposite: feelings of being more isolated, lonely, or trapped in FOMO (fear of missing out). Even the positive posts can cause a tsunami of negative thinking. Do you feel empowered and inspired when you go online, or depressed and depleted? Take a look at your online habits and make your mental health a priority.

I detox from anything that does not support my mental and physical health. I let my body relax into the moment—its natural state. I am my own best friend.

Relaxation Ritual

Turn off all digital screens a few hours before bed and consider doing a digital detox for a few weeks, including removing the apps from your phone.

THE SOURCE OF MY PEACE
IS IN THE RELEASE.

Your body is like a library, storing information from your life, including the emotional results of past experiences and traumas. Body imbalances such as pain and disease can be connected to stores of emotional pain, such as heartache, unprocessed anger, grief, and worries about life.

It's hard to feel harmony when your body is in pain, but you can begin to transform certain imbalances by allowing yourself to feel your feelings. Identify any uncomfortable or painful points in your body, then see if there is a repressed feeling connected to a past experience. The source of your peace is in their release.

I am free of emotional stagnancy and pain.
I feel good in my body and release my aches.
As I feel and process stuck emotions, I am
lighter. This is my path toward harmony.

RELAXATION RITUAL

Identify a painful spot on your body and rub a pain-relieving salve or CBD oil into it. As you lie down to sleep, imagine golden light flooding your body with peaceful intentions. The warm glow of these rays melts away all aches and pains.

I FILL MY MIND WITH NURTURING AND INSPIRING ENERGY.

If you've ever told yourself *I'm not creative* (or *I can't sing* or *I wish I could paint*), consider that the only thing stopping you is your fearful ego that wants to keep you small and manageable. The things you wish you could do but say that you can't are actually areas to explore—think of them as joyful messages from your heart. Not only does engaging in creative projects boost your mental health but it can add immense value to your life, helping you be more present in the moment. (More mindfulness? Yes, please!) It also grows and deepens your skill sets, enriching your life overall.

I take action according to my heart's wise guidance. I find joy in the little things and take great pride in all that I do.

RELAXATION RITUAL

Start expanding your mind in your journal tonight. Write out creative ideas for new expressive outlets that you've always wanted to explore (making pottery, painting, singing, dancing?). Make a plan to do it this week—whatever your heart desires.

I SHARE MY FEELINGS WITH OTHERS AND ALLOW MYSELF TO BE SEEN.

Right now, your emotions may feel overwhelming and isolating—we all have experiences that we feel we cannot share. But you are not alone on your life journey. Give yourself permission to push past the invisible barrier between you and your loved ones, especially when you are struggling. Let them into your inner world by sharing your feelings; when you do, you give them an opportunity to be there for you in ways they never have before. This exchange is a beautiful, supportive process where everyone gets what they truly need.

Feeling and expressing my emotions is part of the human experience. I share this aspect of myself so I can be seen, loved, and supported.

RELAXATION RITUAL

Reach out to a loved one tonight (or this week) and share your feelings around something you're dealing with. (It may be helpful to first ask them if they have bandwidth to listen. Sometimes they don't, and that's okay! Reschedule the call or reach out to someone else you trust.)

I FEEL PROUD OF MYSELF FOR WHAT I ACCOMPLISHED TODAY.

How often do we go through our day without stopping to take note of how much we've done and how far we've actually come? As you wind down and get ready for bed, think about all the amazing things you accomplished today. Feeling proud of yourself is important—you're doing an amazing job! We don't give ourselves enough credit for the things we do daily; our eyes are often set on the end goal, which has yet to be reached. It may seem like celebrating ourselves is selfish or narcissistic, but the opposite is true. When celebrating your successes comes from an intention of love, it is part of honoring yourself and your self-worth.

I am so amazing. I am beautiful. I am divine.
I make it a priority to honor myself—
I am proud to be me.

RELAXATION RITUAL

Bake your favorite cookie recipe tonight to celebrate yourself! As you enjoy your cookies, make a list of the highlights of your day in your journal.

New opportunities come to me because I am whole.

Your self-care journey elevates your energy and brings you back to wholeness.

We are all creators of our own reality, and we cocreate with others because relationships matter. As you encounter others in your life experiences, you always have a choice on where and with whom you want to spend your energy and your time. Moving forward, focus on cocreating a life with those who put good energy and reciprocal attention into your collaborations; align yourself with people who value you, because you value yourself. Do the same with your thoughts and actions. Align your direction with your values, and new opportunities and beginnings will naturally follow.

I am the light and the love that is freely
given to others in the world as well as myself.
I create my reality through my cocreations
and self-alignment. This loving balance is
my strength, for I am whole.

Relaxation Ritual

Before bed, set out your clothes for tomorrow as you look forward to a positive future. What color inspires you? Be sure to include this color in your outfit.

As I relax, all becomes clear.

If you don't take time for adequate self-reflection and rest, you're more likely to act out of unintentional malice, which leads to regret and pain. These are the shadow sides of human nature (the ego dominations) that take hold, especially when you are overworked, stressed, and run-down. It's easier to overreact when your body is not in balance. Tonight, make it an intention to slow down; as you do, things will become clearer—you will no longer see the reactive situations from the same perspective. Take a fresh look at your life from a new perspective to open new realms of possibilities to you.

I prioritize nightly rest for clarity and balance—to live from a heart-centered place. When I rest, I see my life from new perspectives, and I act with wisdom and love.

Relaxation Ritual

Help calm your vagus nerve tonight by dimming or minimizing the light in your bedroom and listening to quiet music before going to bed.

Tension in my body dissipates when I listen to its wisdom.

Do you feel any tightness in your body? Has it been causing you angst or pain? The feeling of tension in your body could be your intuition talking to you. It's possible that these physical messages are from your inner guide, trying to point you toward healing or in a new direction. Perhaps you're in a job that you don't like and you feel restricted; or maybe you're in a relationship where you need to speak up but are afraid to speak your truth. These experiences of holding back can manifest as body ailments that become chronic over time. Honor your body and its messages—there's wisdom in every interaction.

I trust my body and listen to its messages about my inner world. This connection is medicine for my cells and my soul.

Relaxation Ritual

Get into a comfortable position on your bed. Close your eyes and breathe in for five seconds, hold for five seconds, and then release, paying attention to any tightness in your muscles. What is your body's message for you?

I AM OPEN TO UNDERSTANDING.

Any insecurity you have impacts your ability to feel good throughout the day, and this carries over into the night. It doesn't matter how many hours of sleep you get; if you are at war with yourself during the day, it will cause anxiety, stress, and fear well into the night. Be willing to understand the aspects of yourself that you have yet to embrace. Identify sources of self-doubt and be willing to learn more about what is holding you back. Open up to seeing what you have not been able to see before. When you learn to love yourself and appreciate all of who you are, you are boundless—pure love in action.

I am open to understanding more about myself—it allows me to love and care for myself even more. I am stronger and better than I've ever been before.

RELAXATION RITUAL

Tonight, put on your softest pajamas and fluffiest slippers as an act of self-love. Notice how good it feels to be cozy and accepting of yourself in your own body.

I KNOW WHAT I DESERVE FROM THE SACRED LESSONS I HAVE LEARNED.

Your heart is always guiding you in the direction of your highest good, but life can throw you curve balls! Fortunately, when you experience surprises in life, you grow as a person. Tonight is a celebration of all you have learned on your life journey so far. You have gained some valuable lessons that have given you great depth of wisdom, discernment, and a focus on what matters most to you. Know that you deserve this beautiful existence and have earned the right to celebrate the cherished moments of your amazing life.

I listen to my heart and honor my life
experiences. I deserve to be happy,
abundant, and well. I rise into more love
as I allow self-compassion to lift me
into higher vibrations.

RELAXATION RITUAL

Make yourself a cup of your favorite bedtime tea and mindfully enjoy it while reflecting on the best wisdom you've received from a mentor, teacher, or parent.

I DO NOT TAKE EVERYTHING PERSONALLY. IT'S NOT ALWAYS ABOUT ME.

Do you feel you've been wronged, as if something unfair and unjust has recently happened in your life? Trust that whatever is wrong will be made right, but it's not necessarily something you need to focus on. It's important to turn your attention to peace and love for yourself and those around you. You may be hurt right now because of your interpretation of a recent conflict, but do your best not to personalize it. Instead, spend quality time with yourself to reconnect and recalibrate. The most important focus of your life is your life—your sacred, loving relationship with yourself.

My thoughts come and go much like my emotions; I do not attach meaning to either. I let go, trusting that all is in balance and in divine order.

RELAXATION RITUAL

Disconnect from your electronic devices and turn to your journal before bed. Is there anything bothering you that's causing you to overreact? Reconnect inward with love and curiosity to restore your balance.

My intuition is my compass.

If you feel like you have been off track, find yourself distracted from your life purpose, or are wondering why you keep ending up in situations that turn out in the same disappointing way, then it could be because you are failing to trust yourself. Honoring your intuition means trusting the divine inner knowing of your soul. This is your voice of reason; this is the path of truth. Start to realize that your life circumstances can radically change and improve when you stop trusting others over yourself. Always listen to your inner voice first—let it show you the way.

I trust myself daily. In times of distress and need, I go within. My intuition is my guiding light.

Relaxation Ritual

Tonight, get in touch with your intuition through an automatic writing session in your journal. Write nonstop, letting your inner voice have a platform to speak and share. Do not judge, edit, or think about the thoughts; just dive in fully. What is the wisdom that shows up?

WHO I AM IS ENOUGH.

That aspect of yourself that you dislike or are afraid to show others is holding you back from receiving the love that you deserve. You are more than what you do or achieve, what you give, or how much money is in your bank account—none of this has anything to do with your true worth. There's nothing to prove to anyone. Feeling unworthy of receiving the love that you deserve is an old pattern that is ready to be released. Who you are is more than enough.

I am the love that I seek—loving awareness in heart, body, and soul. I have nothing to prove or to become to be worthy. I know my value, and I am enough as I am.

RELAXATION RITUAL

Tonight, meditate and reflect upon a time when you stood up for yourself. Think about how good it felt to have your own back. How can you show up for yourself in the same way this week?

I SEE MYSELF AND THE VALUE I OFFER THE WORLD.

When is the last time you really saw yourself in the way others see you? Most of us do not recognize who we truly are, because we are so hard on ourselves. Whether it's self-criticism, taking care of life to-dos, or focusing on the needs of others, it doesn't take long to feel overworked and exhausted. With so much expended energy it's no surprise you're exhausted. It's easy to forget your inherent goodness when you are tending to all of life's daily demands. Fortunately, when you disengage from the urgency of the outside world to achieve, succeed, and get ahead, you also release yourself from the pressure of external validation. Your inner world is where your value and peace abide. Turn inward and you finally see the stunning being you already are.

I release the need to show the world that I am valuable. Value is not earned; it is already within each of us.

RELAXATION RITUAL

Tonight, as you get ready for bed, take a good look in the mirror as you think to yourself, *I value, love, and respect you.*

I WELCOME MY TEARS AND LET MY FEELINGS FLOW.

Crying can feel awkward at times, especially if you're in front of another person, but tears are valuable gifts we give to ourselves and others. Let yourself cry and express emotions that want to be felt. When your tears come forward, it simply indicates an imbalance within you—your system is trying to find regulation. As you allow the tears to flow, you transcend dense energy to experience more of your true self. Crying is healing—let yourself feel it all. And if you cry in front of another person, there's no need to feel embarrassed; this is a healing experience in itself—a demonstration of sincere vulnerability.

My emotions and tears empower me—
when feelings flow, I fuel my soul.
Authenticity is my strength.

RELAXATION RITUAL

Have a good cry tonight by watching a favorite tear-jerker movie. Conclude the evening with a gentle washing of your face and soothing moisturizer before bed.

I AM COMFORTABLE IN MY LIFE.

As you relax this evening, recognize how comfortable you truly are in your life. So often, we're told we should want more, do more, have more; but the truth is, what you have right now is beautiful, just as it is. You don't need anything else to be happy in this moment.

When you are content, know that it is about being comfortable and happy enough for the time being. Being happy with where you are allows you to appreciate the blessings that are already around you. It's good to feel good; and good can turn into great, especially when we recognize how loved and secure we really are.

It feels good to be in this place and time in my life. I am comfortable and content in my body. I am perfection in this moment— all is well.

RELAXATION RITUAL

Practice getting more comfortable in your own skin with a soothing shower or bath and a gentle body scrub before bed. Fall asleep feeling comfortable and clean.

I AM HERE FOR A REASON. I BELIEVE IN ME.

Tonight is an opportunity to appreciate your family lineage—all your ancestors who have lived before you. You are here because of them, and you are here for a reason. Your family is so proud of you, even if they don't (or can't) show it or have passed on. You have significant things to do in your life on Earth; activating your family's desires for you and clearing ancestral karma is important. Don't ever forget that your life has a purpose, and the healing work you do on yourself heals your family lineage as well.

I trust in my ability to manifest the dreams of my life and all my heart's desires. I know that I am here for a reason, and my ancestors are proud of me.

RELAXATION RITUAL

Before bed, light a candle and send a ripple of appreciation through your familial lines on both sides—gratitude for those who came before you and for your life now. (Just make sure to blow out the candle before going to sleep.)

I CONNECT TO MY HEART AND SET MYSELF FREE.

As you wind down and enter deeper into your evening, connect to your heart—that central force that is always with you, offering guidance, inspiration, and support. When you drop into your heart and lead with love, you start to see through the illusions and the mental gymnastics that the ego pursues and projects; you experience less chaos and confusion. Free yourself from stress by dropping into your inner world. The guidance from your heart will always lead you to freedom.

I connect inward, with my heart, to free myself from stress and worry. This moment is important, for I have an opportunity to be one with all that exists. I see my life with clarity as I free myself from all illusions.

RELAXATION RITUAL

Before you fall asleep tonight, place your hands on your heart chakra and breathe in the love of the universe—that love that is meant just for you, exactly as you are.

I SHAPE MY IDENTITY. I AM SAFE.

Sometimes, we feel hurt and misunderstood, especially when others do something unknowingly that triggers anxious, unsettled feelings from our past. The mother wound (feelings of abandonment) and father wound (feelings of not being protected) can recur in adulthood, especially if the original traumas never healed.[29] As children, if our needs were not met by our parents or caretakers, we may continue to feel unsafe in the world as adults—an internalized belief that you can't trust others, which shaped part of your identity. But *you* are your own best provider and protector now—you don't need to look further than yourself.

I take responsibility for my healing, providing what I need to feel secure in my life. I protect myself with patience, love, and care.

RELAXATION RITUAL

Before bed, take a warm bath or shower with a few drops of lavender or jasmine essential oil mixed with a little almond or jojoba oil. Think about or imagine a happy childhood memory when you felt protected, cared for, and loved.

I EMBRACE THE SEASON OF MY SOUL.

Peace is your purpose, and serenity is your birthright; however, it may not always feel this way, especially when you are in transition. Just like the seasons of nature, we have seasons for our souls. When you move from one season and grow into the next, there is often a period of unknown. Unfortunately, the unknown can be a time of fear for many, but it doesn't have to be. Embrace these changes and their growing pains—they lead to new beginnings. You are endlessly expansive, and better things are always coming your way.

I leave the old behind and embrace the new—I trust the process of my expansion. As I tap deeper into the moment, I am serene and calm.

RELAXATION RITUAL

Before bed, close your eyes and envision one of your favorite places in nature and imagine the seasons transitioning into your favorite one. Relax in this serene environment as you visualize nature shifting into more peace in your imagination.

I AM EMOTIONALLY MATURE AND IN CONTROL OF MY REACTIONS.

Your feelings are knocking at your door. If you're avoiding feeling them, the knocking will only become louder and more intense. And if you don't allow yourself to feel your feelings regularly, they can become tsunamis of dysregulation, overpowering you and those around you with intense reactions. If you've ever been called dramatic or too sensitive, it's possible your emotions were disturbing your peace. Being sensitive is not a bad thing, nor is it a weakness to feel things deeply. But learning how to control your emotions is essential to staying grounded and balanced.

My emotions are my guides, not my drivers.
I am the master of my reactions and in
control of my life.

RELAXATION RITUAL

What are you feeling tonight? Use your journal to get in touch with yourself by identifying your feelings using "I" statements (i.e., "I feel nervous") and then try to articulate why ("I feel nervous because . . ."). There is no need to react to your feelings, simply allow them to come and go. Conclude this practice with love and gratitude for the insights these emotions provided.

I ALLOW MYSELF TO RELEASE PARTS OF ME I DON'T IDENTIFY WITH ANYMORE.

Life operates on a vibrational timeline—one that is aligned to your highest good. When elements of your character, personality, and lifestyle no longer fit with the direction you are meant to go, the timeline shifts and those things that no longer serve you fall away. Even when the changes are motivated by exciting events, you may still need to grieve the loss of the old aspects of your life. Recognize how you have evolved and changed; you can't be the person you were before even if you tried. Let this shedding of the old inspire and support you as you embrace your life from a new, authentic place.

Who I was yesterday led to who I am today.
I recognize the wisdom that comes from my
past experiences and embrace each evolution
in my life.

RELAXATION RITUAL

Detox your sleep space. Is your nightstand cluttered with unnecessary items? Is the lighting harsh? Do two things tonight to make your bedroom more inviting and remove what you no longer identify with anymore.

I AM COMFORTABLE SPENDING TIME DOING WHAT I LOVE.

What aspects of yourself do you absolutely love? Do you have a passion or a hobby you keep secret? Sometimes we hide the parts of ourselves that we love in order to protect them—we're afraid they won't be well received by others. Perhaps you have a goal that you're afraid to share. When you go to bed tonight, think about how much joy this love of yours brings you, and invite more of it into your life. Give yourself permission to share yourself by expressing your joy through expressing your passion.

I activate the deepest aspects of myself and shine brightly with grace and joy. I nurture the parts of myself that I absolutely love, and I freely share these aspects with others.

RELAXATION RITUAL

Tonight, charge your amethyst crystal (great for inspiring creativity) by placing it on a windowsill, under the moonlight. Place it under your pillow before bed to welcome your new era of creativity and self-expression.

I VIEW ALL SITUATIONS THROUGH THE LENS OF LOVE AND LIGHT.

Loving another is not always an unconditional experience; it's human nature to put conditions on our love. We need others to be a certain way for us to give our love, but learning how to live from an unconditional, loving space is part of your expanded spiritual journey. Let go of the need for people to give you something or act in a specific way by first being more loving to yourself. Are you waiting for another person to be more kind, generous, or warm before you open yourself to them? Start by being the love you seek. Unconditional love transmutes worry and fear.

I open myself to giving and receiving unconditional love. I learn from situations that require me to practice being more loving. I begin by loving myself.

RELAXATION RITUAL

Do something tonight to make someone's day this week. Write a handwritten note to a person you appreciate. Consider how they have extended love and acceptance to you and thank them for it.

WITH EACH BREATH, I CHOOSE PEACE AND CALM.

It's hard to fall asleep when your mind keeps working through problems, trying to solve situations that don't need to be solved in that moment. Dissipate these anxieties through your breath and choosing to be in the present— *now* is the time for rest and sleep. Before you even head for your bedroom, begin focusing on calm presence and the quality of your breath. Breathe slowly in and out of your body, feeling the oxygen flow into your diaphragm and then into your lungs, expanding them; focus on the same as you exhale. Drift deeper into the evening, and fall asleep with the mindset that all is well.

I surrender my thoughts and worries.
I am in the moment, and peace is my reality.
My breath brings loving awareness and calm.

RELAXATION RITUAL

Make yourself into a blanket burrito to fall asleep. Use the blankets to wrap yourself in a giant hug, embraced in warmth and comfort. Continue to focus on the quality of your breath, breathing deeply and freely, knowing that you are safe.

I LET GO OF MY NEED TO CONTROL THE OUTCOME.

You've been putting enormous pressure on yourself lately. Are you working to reach a big goal but feel like you're pushing yourself past capacity? Are you trying to make sure that everything meets your expectations? The outcome is not something that you can control, and the attempt to do so is exhausting, making it impossible to feel balanced at night. Look at all your priorities—what is taking most of your energy? In what area are you feeling burned out? It's time to surrender to the process and let go of the outcome. You don't need to control anything. Know you're right where you need to be in this journey.

I release my need for a specific outcome.
I surrender all expectations. I trust the
process—everything happens for a reason.

RELAXATION RITUAL

Lie on your back in bed. Breathe in deeply and then exhale an intentional sigh of relief, making a humming sound. Allow the sound to release all the way through you, from your head to your toes.

I FOCUS ON THE GOOD THINGS ALL AROUND ME.

Everything in our life does not have to be good, and every day does not have to be great. There's already an enormous amount of pressure to show up fully to do the work, to be happy, to achieve, to succeed, but this is not the reality of the human experience. There are some days when it's hard to make it through, and it's okay to admit this. Find comfort in the good things that are all around you. Even if you don't feel good right now, this is not about spiritual bypassing; it's about appreciating the small things, even when things feel hard. Tonight, focus on what is going well, and release the day's challenges with love.

I appreciate my life and everything that is going well. I understand the human experience is wide and vast, and I am present for each moment.

RELAXATION RITUAL

Tonight, sit in silence and connect to the power of *now*. Do nothing—just *be!* Allow yourself to be in your own company and enjoy how good it feels.

With each experience, I'm growing and learning.

While it is important to appreciate what is going well in life, continue to look at your blind spots too; don't avoid what still needs improvement. It may feel like the pillars that hold up your life structure will become unbalanced if you do, but looking at the shadow side of yourself is healthy and necessary for growth.

Take some time for self-awareness, illuminating the areas of your life that you have ignored. How can you become stronger and more resilient in these areas? Be fully transparent and honest with yourself by making choices that align with your integrity and values.

I am always expanding and growing—
when I learn, I grow past what I knew before.
I accept these opportunities to participate
fully in my life.

Relaxation Ritual

Make time for self-awareness before bed. Massage your temples as you focus on a recent experience and the resilience it took to be where you are now. Identify the lessons you learned from it and offer gratitude for how you've grown.

THE RIGHT PATH ALWAYS APPEARS.

Do you have a big life decision that you're trying to make? Are you in transition and wondering which path to choose? The right direction always appears when you align with what vibrationally matches your values. It would be great to see the whole picture to know the outcome, but the truth is, you can only take one step at a time. As you connect to your heart and identify with what is most important, you will never be led astray. All you have to do is surrender to the moment, right here and now. Trust what is unfolding just for you, because you are provided for and dearly loved.

No choice is wrong, for all my choices bring clarity. I choose what aligns with my heart.

RELAXATION RITUAL

Light a candle and sit in silence as you mediate on a big decision you've been struggling with lately. What does your inner wisdom tell you about this? Release the need to force the answers; the truth will come in the silence as you look to the light.

I RELEASE MY GRIEF AND LEARN THE LESSONS IN LOVE.

Whether you're healing from a recent life change, breakup, job loss, or betrayal, acknowledging your grief is essential. Everyone experiences loss in their own way, and mourning is an important part of the process. Healing takes time— months, even years—but for some people, prolonged grief takes its toll. When we grieve, we are learning the lessons associated with giving of our heart—this is true love. We are here on Earth to learn lessons in love even if it is through loss. If you grieve and have ruminating thoughts, recognize there is power in this process. Studies show that failure to reconcile conflict can prolong grief.[30] If there are any con- flicts or unresolved issues affecting your healing, amend the situation. Grief, too, is a means of learning and evolving.

I realize grief is a form of learning, and I give the process the time that it needs. I do not have any regrets.

RELAXATION RITUAL

Commune with your ancestors this week by preparing one of their favorite meals. Make a list and a plan in your journal before bed. Consider inviting a guest to share in this honor of your loved one.

I SET THE STANDARDS FOR MY LIFE.

Wanting to be seen in a certain light prevents you from shining your authentic light. Don't strive to fit into a box that others deem right for you. It's your life; you get to make the rules and set the standards. When people say things about you that you know are not true, recognize it is a perception from their own experience. As you fall asleep tonight, focus on the peace that resides inside of you. All is well as it is. Free yourself from the need for approval from the outside world.

Peace—my point of purpose—is within me at all times. I choose to abide by my truth—the light and love that I am. I release my need to belong to the outside world, for I belong to myself.

RELAXATION RITUAL

Color in a coloring book tonight. Feel free to color outside the lines or to use multiple colors where you'd normally use only one. Use this opportunity to have fun according to your own rules.

I EMBRACE THE GENTLE ASPECTS OF MY NATURE.

The divine feminine lives within all of us—a force that is not about gender but the energy of our nurturing, supportive, grounding, and healing aspects. You have a side of yourself that wants to be nurtured more. Focus on your softer qualities—those that are graceful, relaxed, and gentle. You don't have to work so hard or hustle to make your way through life. You'll know you've been living too much in your masculine energy when you are stressed, overwhelmed, and exhausted. Find balance by stepping deeper into your feminine energy. Rest, allowing yourself to just *be*. Nurture this moment as it *is*, not as you think it should be.

I release my need to strive for more than what is. I stop and let myself be. I am relaxed and secure as I am.

RELAXATION RITUAL

Throw yourself a dance party before bed. Play a few of your favorite songs, moving your body wherever the music takes you. Free yourself from restriction and judgment, and just have fun!

I AM IN THE HIGHEST SERVICE TO OTHERS WHEN I FOCUS ON MY HEALING.

Everyone is operating from their own level of awareness, doing the best they can with what they know and have been taught. To transcend our darker aspects, we must recognize the power of healing; when we heal, we do better—we evolve. You are in a place in your life where healing is essential to the advancement of your soul; this is the path of highest service to others. Instead of thinking something is wrong with you or blaming yourself and others, go on a healing journey and commit to doing the work.

As I release the burdens of past pain, I free myself energetically. I ascend into the next phase of my life and my ability to serve others.

RELAXATION RITUAL

Do a wellness check-in tonight. Lay down in the coziest place in your home, close your eyes, and scan your body. Tighten and relax each muscle, reflecting on inner shifts and alignment. Send compassion and breath to any stuck areas until you feel more grounded.

I AM NO LONGER AFRAID OF CHANGE.

One thing is certain: change is inevitable. And change can be incredibly difficult and uncomfortable, especially when it feels forced upon us from work, family, and the outside world. Learn how to navigate the stages of your life by being open to change—it will feel much more relaxed. When we fear and resist change, it's often because we are holding on to the past; we haven't given ourselves permission to fully embrace where we want to go. Instead of letting change happen to you, focus on being intentional by creating the life you truly want.

I embrace change, for I am being guided into new possibilities. I am free of worry as I welcome my next chapter—it is aligned with my highest good.

RELAXATION RITUAL

Get ready for bed early by getting out of your daytime (work) clothes and changing into something more comfortable. Designate a "relaxation" outfit tonight to signal your brain that it's time to relax whenever you put it on.

My body feels weightless and peaceful.

The heaviness you feel in your body could be worry, stress, frustration, or pain; but it could also be other people's burdens that have been energetically dumped onto you. You give people permission to attach or detach with the boundaries you set. You may not realize that when you are there for others by listening and offering advice, their pain can attach itself to you, especially if you are an empath or sensitive soul. Allow people to have their own experiences, but protect your energy too. When you do, you'll feel buoyant in your body, free of carrying any burdens that are not yours.

I have strong boundaries—I am there for others but do not take on their pain as my own. I am light in my energy and light in my thoughts. I am weightless in my body, for I am at peace.

Relaxation Ritual

Practice protection and boundaries in your sacred sleep space. Use a blue-light filter on your phone and laptop tonight to see if you feel more rested in the morning.

MY BODY IS FREE OF STRAIN.

We hold our emotions as energetic pockets throughout our body, and this eventually builds up as tension. Are you feeling particularly uncomfortable in your neck and shoulders? Your back? Your hips? Release your stress by breathing into these pockets—it's one of the best ways to relax your muscles. Prioritize body bliss through an activating relaxation session, giving your mind and body dedicated time to acknowledge and release this tension. Free yourself of worry and pain one breath and one muscle at a time.

My body is gorgeous and healthy and alive—
I celebrate all that it does for me.
I free it from stress and pain through
daily care and rest.

RELAXATION RITUAL

Before bed, make a cup of tea and drink it mindfully. Pay attention to the sensations in your body as you sip your tea: Is there an experience or a memory connected to them? Gently process and release the emotions with your breath as you drink in self-compassion.

TODAY IS A GIFT. I REST IN APPRECIATION.

Getting a great night of sleep starts first thing in the morning—what you think, feel, eat, drink, and do sets you up for the entire day. Being intentional about your choices in the morning helps you feel more grounded and calm in the hours that follow. When you relax in the evening and prepare for sleep, you will be able to rest easier when you've had a good day prior. Everything is connected in your life, from the moment you wake to the moment you close your eyes again. Tonight, celebrate your day to set yourself up for a good sleep and a great tomorrow.

I am blessed beyond measure. I wake up and I fall asleep with gratitude for a life well lived.

RELAXATION RITUAL

Use your time before bed to create a mindful morning routine. Develop a short list of activities that make you feel empowered. Write it down, put it in a prominent place (perhaps your bathroom mirror), and stick to it for the next week.

EVERY CELL IN MY BODY IS IN PERFECT ORDER.

Stress impacts every part of your body, including your cells. Your cells have needs too—they work hard to keep your body in optimal order. When you feel aches and pains, this is a signal that something is out of balance within—your body has a message for you. Your cells want you to know that they love you and desire to keep you healthy, but they need rest and care to do this. Don't work yourself so hard that your body cannot rest. When you get sufficient sleep, your entire body thrives.

I breathe in oxygen and send it to all my cells. I celebrate the well-being of my entire body. I rest to show my body that I care for it. I appreciate every cell and its contribution to wholeness. I am at peace.

RELAXATION RITUAL

Water plays a big part in replenishing cells, so hydrate! Drink a big glass of filtered water as you wind down for the night. (Alkaline water is the best option.)

I ENJOY OPTIMAL HEALTH AND VIBRANT ENERGY.

Having vibrant, reliable energy is the ultimate goal, and having a routine for quality sleep helps you reach it. So often, we think about a wellness routine through the lens of fitness or nutrition, but make sure you're adding in stress-relief and mental-health activities. Focus on self-care rituals each day and night. Your health is not just your physical appearance or what you eat; it is what you think, what you do, and how you rest your body and mind. Give yourself more energy tomorrow by relaxing and slowing down tonight, at least several hours before bed. When you slow down, you give yourself the energy you need to maintain optimum wellness.

I take care of myself with rest, prioritizing quality sleep. I wake refreshed, with the vibrant energy I need to thrive.

RELAXATION RITUAL

Focus on doing something tonight that will make your morning easier, such as prepping your breakfast, packing your lunch, or setting out your clothes. Prepare your body for rest by winding down earlier and relieving those first to-dos tomorrow.

I SEE BLESSINGS EVERYWHERE.

It can be hard to feel like the world has any good in it when there is so much pain for so many, but this is an opportunity to look at an unjust situation from a new lens. Most people are trying to survive and do the best they can, but sometimes, it comes from a place of lack and fear. You don't have to live your life from this lower vibration, however. Remember that those who hurt you in life are hurting inside. This is no excuse for abusive and bad behavior, but instead of hurting them back, rise above the situation. See this as a blessing for you to practice and to be more loving.

I choose to see everything through the lens of love. I am aligned to divine love, and my self-love is strong.

RELAXATION RITUAL

Raise your vibration tonight by avoiding high-fat and processed foods, sugar, and caffeine at least three hours before bedtime. Your body and your sleep will thank you.

It's not mine to worry about.

It's time to free yourself from the situation that has been causing you the most pain—there's no need for you to think about it anymore. The universe is asking you to free your mind, especially from the worries of the past. When you stay stuck there, even in your mind, you prevent new opportunities from coming to you. Give yourself permission to enter a new phase of your life. Future opportunities are waiting for you with open arms! The more you worry about the past, the less freedom you have to move forward into a more joyful, happy state. A new life and peaceful space awaits.

I free myself from all worry, guilt, and heaviness from the past. Everything that happened has helped me become who I am meant to be, and I am grateful.

Relaxation Ritual

Bring out your journal before bed and reflect on what the next new phase of your life will be like. What you are looking forward to, and how does this make you feel?

101

I HAVE THE COURAGE TO GO DEEPER INTO MY HEART.

It takes courage to live from your heart and make choices that feel aligned with your true self, especially when there's a lot of pressure from those around you to do what they think is best. When you're in conflict with others, it can be hard to rest, for you do not have inner peace. Be still with yourself and listen to the quiet voice within. Before you make a sudden move, take some time to reflect on the situations that need attention. Go into your heart and listen to its guidance on how to best move forward. It will never take you off course.

I have the courage to live fully from my heart.
I listen to its guidance, and I let it lead
me into harmonious unions with
others and myself.

RELAXATION RITUAL

As a bedtime treat, grab your favorite oversized mug and fill it with hot chocolate, cocoa, or cacao (which is heart open-ing). As you sip this comforting drink, feel the warmth of gratitude fill your heart.

I SEE THE TRUTH AS IT IS, WITHOUT JUDGMENT.

Everybody has their own version of truth, for everyone is operating from their own perspectives, beliefs, and opinions. What is one person's truth is not another's, yet every truth can exist for each person. It's important to respect others and what they feel is right for them, but it's more important for you to listen to *your* inner truth. Your voice within is wise beyond your physical years. Allow people to believe what they believe, and focus on the truth that aligns to you. In the end, truth always prevails, whether we like what it has to say or not. Let the honesty of what is real for you guide you forward.

I honor and trust myself and do what is aligned with love. I see the truth in all situations, without judgment, relaxing into the comfort of its wisdom.

RELAXATION RITUAL

Create your own relaxing aromatherapy spray by mixing water or rose water and a few drops of your favorite essential oil in a spray bottle. Spritz on your pillows and bedding before bed.

My kindness is a superstrength.

Love is understanding and patient. It's also forgiving—but not at the detriment of self. Some believe kindness is a form of weakness, but those who think this way are usually operating from a place of unresolved pain and low self-worth. On the contrary, kindness is a sign of incredible strength. It's particularly important to recognize this when you are in a situation where it is hard to forgive. Be patient with yourself—don't force forgiveness. Practice kindness and love with yourself first to heal the hurts within. In due time, forgiveness will happen.

My kindness is a strength that makes me stronger. I work to forgive myself and others, as this kindness adds to my strength and theirs.

Relaxation Ritual

Tonight, take a piece of paper and write a letter to someone from your past who has hurt you and you've had a difficult time forgiving. You don't have to send the letter (unless you want to); just let yourself say what you are still holding on to inside. Put the letter in an envelope for safekeeping, then release (during the next full moon) its contents with love.

I AM THE SOURCE OF MY ABUNDANCE.

Choosing to be in an abundant mindset instead of a scarcity mindset is a choice we make every moment. When you feel yourself falling into fear and worry, go inward and feel the abundance there—its radiance can uplift you and others. Tonight, focus on bringing more love to yourself, starting from the inside. Feel gratitude for your beating heart and your beautiful body and mind. Celebrate yourself as the one-of-a-kind person you are—there's no one else like you! Feel the abundance of your body and the life it allows you to manifest.

I tap into the amazing energy of abundance within me and let it lead me forward to opportunity, prosperity, and fulfillment. Its positive life force flows through me effortlessly.

RELAXATION RITUAL

Tonight, as you lay yourself down to sleep, meditate on what the most abundant aspect of your life is right now and appreciate it fully. Gratitude creates more abundance.

I DESERVE TO SAVOR LIFE'S JOYFUL MOMENTS.

You don't have to live a jam-packed life to have a good one. Throughout the day, it's easy to race through each task and overlook the important, simple moments that could bring us joy. Pleasure comes in the moments we savor; joy exists in the times between where you were and where you're trying to go—in the present. If you're working hard in life and trying to succeed, you can miss the moments of opportunity that are here, right now. Tonight, relax more so you can refresh yourself. When you do, you will create more moments of joy.

I activate joy by relaxing and celebrating myself. I take time for me, recognizing the happiness in simple yet powerful moments of presence.

RELAXATION RITUAL

For tonight's bedtime snack, grab a small piece of chocolate (or favorite decadent treat) and engage all your senses in the study of it: how does it smell, look, feel in your mouth, taste, affect your mood? Be intentional—don't rush through any of the senses.

It's okay to take a break.

There is no need to push ahead so hard. As you take time to reflect upon your day, pause in the present moment, giving your body and mind time and space to restore themselves. Restoration is an important part of your healing process and personal well-being. When we think of personal development, we often think of maintaining a proper mindset or of achieving goals and new growth, but today, consider rest as your biggest goal and achievement. When you take a break, you have the energy to move forward with balance and focus.

I rest gently yet fiercely—my power is in the pause. I step fully into my life only after a time of adequate recovery and rejuvenation. I prioritize relaxation every day.

Relaxation Ritual

Take a mental break by studying your bedroom, looking for something soothing to your tired body, mind, and spirit, such as a plant or a picture. Once you find it, gaze at it for a few moments with no purpose beyond this calm connection.

I FEEL EVERY PART OF ME RELAXING.

When you go to bed at night, which position do you naturally fall into? The way you sleep—on your stomach, back, or side—makes a difference to your physical and mental health each day. If you wake up with body aches, headaches, or pain, it could be your position at night. If you sleep with someone else in the bed (including a pet), this can also cause disruptions, like snoring and restlessness. Make an intention to consciously pay attention to your sleep positions and situation, and shift them as needed to establish more harmony and optimal rest.

I fall deeper into the experience of relaxation, and I am at ease. I close my eyes and feel the sensations of peace as my body becomes lighter. I am safe in this sacred space.

RELAXATION RITUAL

Dim or turn off any harsh lights for a few hours before bed, using this as a signal to start connecting to your own warm energy and inner light, with less effort and distraction.

I DETACH AND ALLOW THINGS TO BE AS THEY ARE. I ACCEPT WHAT IS.

Disengage from the frantic, chaotic energy happening throughout the day. Whether you have a difficult work situation or you're arguing with a loved one, it's time to detach and let the situation be as it is. Surrender yourself to the moment by turning off your mind and turning away from the difficulty. As you transition from the hectic day into the night, go out into nature to get some fresh air. This change of energy flow always helps to get a new perspective on any situation.

I let go of stressful situations and refresh my energy with fresh air. I detach from the worry and anxiety tied to unknown outcomes. I surrender fully, listening to my body and its wisdom, and trusting the process.

RELAXATION RITUAL

To refresh the energy of your sleeping space, open a bedroom window before bedtime and let the fresh air come in for a few minutes. Leave the window open all night if it's comfortable to do so.

My emotions are an expression, not a direction.

Having emotional stability means that your emotions don't control you—you are in charge of regulating your emotions. There's an area of your life where your emotions have overtaken your experience of a situation and clouded your perspective. Perhaps you have overreacted from a place of fear. Outbursts of emotions indicate that you are not allowing yourself to feel them regularly or fully when you do. This is an opportunity to pay attention to your inner world and emotional landscape. Let yourself be present with your emotions, recognizing them as your guides, not your leaders.

I express my emotions without allowing them to take over—I am in charge. I use my emotions to monitor and care for my inner landscape.

Relaxation Ritual

Draw a warm bubble bath before bed, adding several drops of lavender essential oil mixed with a tablespoon of carrier oil, like almond or jojoba (optional) to the water. As you unwind your mind and body, get curious about your emotional landscape, identifying where emotions live in your body and why.

I LET OTHERS BE WHO THEY ARE, NOT WHO I NEED THEM TO BE.

Recognizing that other people have their own needs, behaviors, and perspectives is very important to healthy relationships. Sometimes we find ourselves involved in situations where we are trying to get other people to do or think what we think they should, but we are only seeing their life from our perspective. Allowing them to be who they are is a form of support and love. It's not your job to fix, force, or change anyone. Trust that others are right where they're supposed to be.

I let others be who they inherently are,
allowing them to share the gift of their
unique inner world. I do this as an act of love
and support for them as well as myself.

RELAXATION RITUAL

Unwind with a loved one before bed. Call a friend or family member to practice active listening with them. Don't try to change, fix, or solve their problems; just be there for them and bask in the connection you share.

I AM NOT TOO LATE. ANYTHING MEANT FOR ME WILL NEVER PASS ME BY.

Do you feel that what you've wanted so often in life feels off track, especially with society's invisible benchmarks? Whether it's having a degree, a house, a marriage, or children, all the pressure can pile up. The reality is that you are on your own journey—you have your own life path to walk. It could look completely different from anything around you. Honor this path and free yourself from meeting the expectations of the world. You are not late. There are no worries about getting older. Everything that is meant for you will never pass you by.

I am aligned to my true self, and from this place, all is possible. I do not need to compare myself to others—I am not off track or behind. Right where I am is divine.

RELAXATION RITUAL

Do some intuitive drawing on a sketch pad before bed. Intuitive drawing is simply drawing whatever comes to mind. Enjoy the process of the path that unfolds.

I NOTICE MY TRIGGERS AND STAY CONSCIOUS OF THEM.

Think about a trigger you've recently experienced. What happened? Where did you feel it in your body? Triggers are caused by unhealed wounds from our past that cause an intense emotional reaction in the present. To become more conscious of your whole-body experience, understand that there is an emotional attachment to the experience that feels similar to what you're going through now. Identify the feeling by asking yourself, *When was the first time I felt this way?* Understanding the origin of your trigger starts you on the path toward healing.

> I understand that when I am triggered, it is because there is something that I need to heal from my past. I am conscious of my triggers, and I am not defined by my emotional attachments or reaction to them.

RELAXATION RITUAL

Tonight, as you lie comfortably in bed, identify a recent trigger that caused you to have an emotional outburst. Focus on where you felt it in your body—that space where the trigger was activated—and send it love.

Peaceful energy surrounds me.

An angelic experience cultivates peace all around you. This energy is always available but easily clouded by drama and illusions. There is no need to stay stuck in chaos when peace is available to you. Lean into this angelic support—it is always offering protection and support; you just have to ask for help. If you feel alone, rest assured: you are not, for love surrounds you in every moment. It is here right now and ready to be activated. All you have to do is choose to be in peace and welcome in the loving vibrations.

Peaceful energy is all around and within me. Angels love me and are here for me. They want the best for me, and I ask them for help when I need it.

Relaxation Ritual

Put on an eye mask over your eyes and rest your body in bed. Allow yourself to focus on peace, imagining your guardian angel loving and protecting you as you fall sleep.

When things feel uncertain, I focus on my faith.

Uncertainty exists when we don't have full faith in the big picture, and it can make daily life difficult. This energy does not serve you, clogging up your aura. When we do not trust ourselves or lean into what we know is real, the unreal (the space in between where you are and where you want to go) becomes the focus—an illusion of fear. Take this opportunity to have faith in the highest outcome and the best opportunity for all involved; there's no need to focus on what is not going well. Turn your attention to the possibilities of things working out in your favor.

*I am focused on the moment and my faith.
I direct my energy to the strength of my
convictions. I release fear on the cellular
level and replace it with love.*

Relaxation Ritual

While sitting up in bed, place one hand on your heart and the other on your belly, and close your eyes. Breathe in love and breathe out fear, until your body relaxes fully.

I BREATHE TO RELEASE TENSION AND RETURN TO TRANQUILITY.

Your breath is a tool that you can activate at any moment to release tension. As you go deeper into your evening routine, consciously focus on the quality of your breath: is it short and shallow (tense) or deep and replenishing (relaxed)? Let your breath be the leader into the evening—the medicine that heals your body. Oxygen is a powerful healing elixir you can access at any moment to help you reach calm. It activates your cells with positive vibrations as you replenish them with intentional care.

I breathe into pockets of discomfort with oxygen and loving energy. The medicine of my breath is the gift I can give my body at any time.

RELAXATION RITUAL

As you fall asleep, let the calm sensation of wellness wash over you as you consciously breathe more focused and deeply. Visualize the cells in your body being pumped full of oxygen as they glow with good health.

I AM CAPABLE BEYOND MEASURE.

You've only scratched the surface of what you are able to do in this life. You may feel like you've done all you can and have hit your endpoint, whether it be with a project, dream, relationship, career endeavor, or life benchmark. You feel enough is enough, but this is an opportunity to fall into a deeper state of rest and resurface with more energy and conscious flow. You're capable of so much more than you realize or have allowed. For tonight, retreat, rest, and go into a deep evening of replenishment. As you fall asleep, think about the wonderful possibilities of your life and your future.

I am connected to my highest self—the highest potential available to me. I activate my ideas and goals, and focus fully on possibilities. I feel capable and expansive.

RELAXATION RITUAL

It's time to refresh your sleeping space. Change your sheets or rearrange the furniture, and fall into bed tonight with appreciation for all the wonderful possibilities in your life.

My mind and body work together.

Your mind dictates the direction of your life with your thoughts. Since we manifest first in the realm of our imagination, our thoughts become experiences grounded in reality the more we focus on them. Are you thinking on the stresses of the day or the peaceful close of it? Let your imagination and mind guide you into a state of relaxation this evening. Your body will respond as your mind directs your thoughts into a serene state. Manifest a beautiful night's sleep by focusing the intention of good rest in your mind first.

My mind is my source of inspiration as it guides me into a deeper state of relaxation. I use my thoughts to direct my life into calm and peaceful situations. My body is relaxed, and I fall asleep with ease.

RELAXATION RITUAL

Clear all the energetic heavy energy in preparation for sleep. Hold a quartz crystal in your hand and wave it around to refresh your space. Then meditate on serenity and calm as you clear and balance your body and mind.

I AM COMMITTED TO MY GROWTH AND ITS POSITIVE IMPACT ON THE WORLD.

Laws of karma govern all of life and its forces. Abiding by them unlocks a more fulfilled and aligned life. One of the karmic laws is that of growth. Many people try to control, manipulate, and dominate others, but we have no agency over anyone or anything; we are all sovereign beings. If you have been feeling controlled or have been controlling of others, invite this law back into your life, bringing your attention back to you. To positively impact the world, you can only focus on and change your own growth.

I am in control of my own actions and choose to focus on my own growth. A sense of balance washes over me when I commit to positively impacting the world.

RELAXATION RITUAL

As you focus on something blue in your bedroom, imagine a blue wave of calm and relaxation pouring over your body. Start with your head and let the calm and relaxation flow slowly downward to your feet, removing all tension as it goes.

I LET GO OF WHAT I DO NOT NEED.

Have you been spending your time energetically focusing on helping others with a situation that is theirs to solve? It's beautiful that you want to help, but this puts constraints on your energy and theirs as well. You don't need to help others at the expense of yourself; you can be there for them without having to solve their problems. There is no need to participate in problems that aren't yours. Let yourself feel free by removing yourself from everything that does not serve you and bringing your focus back to yourself.

I focus my energy on myself to feel stronger and more connected to what is true and real for me. I support others best when I allow them to solve their problems and I take charge of my own.

RELAXATION RITUAL

Tonight, reflect in your journal on a time when you tried to help someone but, in hindsight, realize it would have been better to stay out of it. How would you do things differently next time?

All my experiences help me to grow.

Take a moment to put a hand on your heart and thank yourself for your courage and resilience. You have risen above the turbulence! Your experiences have helped you grow into a more expansive version of you, demonstrating a strength larger than life. Let this warrior energy set you free.

Use tonight as a reminder that you don't have to work so hard moving forward. Relax knowing that no matter what life throws at you, you're going to be okay. You are blessed because of the strength in your heart and your strong mental mindset. Stand tall and feel proud of the growth you have experienced.

I am the victor, not the victim. Every trial and tribulation makes me stronger. My resilience is a strength that I hold dear to my heart.

Relaxation Ritual

Settle in tonight by evoking the warrior energy inside your body. Activate your third-eye energy (intuition) by doing an EFT (emotional freedom technique) tapping exercise in the spot between your eyebrows on your forehead.[31]

I RISE WHEN EVERYTHING HEAVY FALLS AWAY.

It's time for you to care for yourself and let the heavy energy of the day fall away. Just like when you get a wonderful massage or Reiki session, the dense energy can blissfully fall away from your current experience. Clear your energy and move away from density by simply focusing on your intention to do so. Heaviness lives in your body, but it doesn't have to indefinitely. Free yourself by consciously making the choice: *I let all dense energy fall away with grace and ease.*

I let go of the heavy energy of fear and worry. I have done my part and shown up the best that I can. I release everything that weighs down my spirit.

RELAXATION RITUAL

Cleanse your energy field before you go to bed by motioning your hands over your body, literally brushing off all unnecessary energy. Flick away the heaviness. Brush your hands across every part of your body, from your head and shoulders to your chest, stomach, knees, and toes.

I COMMUNICATE WITH HONESTY AND A WILLINGNESS TO CONNECT.

Body language, unspoken words, and masking true intentions are all forms of illusion or a hidden agenda when it comes to communication, connection, and trust. Communication is one of the most valuable ways to bridge misunderstandings and develop intimacy. When we say one thing but do another, hide our true feelings, or say what we think another person wants to hear, we deceive them as well as ourselves. Living authentically starts from the inside—a direct expression of the peace and harmony of our inner world. Any discord there will manifest on the outside, too, challenging our ability to communicate freely.

I bless and release the emotional barriers between myself and those closest to me. I choose stability over fear, intimacy over isolation. My personal landscape is at peace, inside and out.

RELAXATION RITUAL

Before bed, practice stretching your trust boundaries by sharing something personal with a loved one. You can journal on what you will say first or speak directly to them. Tell them how much they mean to you.

I GIVE MYSELF CREDIT FOR ALL THAT I AM.

The moon is comfortable in all her phases—she does not race to the next one, allowing rest in each phase with full acceptance for what is. Likewise, there is no need for you to be in another place right now; settle into and surrender to this moment.

Our anxious minds rush to the future or revisit the past—the ego's sneaky way of keeping you from your divine power and connection to self, both of which only live in the present moment. Allow yourself to manifest from this place of alignment and true knowing. Give yourself full access to your inner power and rest in your beautiful light.

I am illuminated with love and the freedom to be me. I live in the present and rest deep in my being as I allow myself to be who I truly am.

RELAXATION RITUAL

Tonight, use the bright moon's energy (go outside, to a window, or use your mind's eye) to illuminate any shadow beliefs or worries, then hand them over to the moon with love and finality.

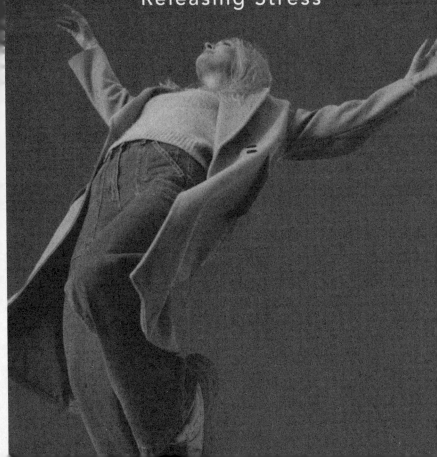

2

Bedtime Mantras for Releasing Stress

I MAKE DECISIONS EASILY WHEN I AM ALIGNED WITH MY HIGHER SELF.

Tonight, give yourself permission to look at any over-whelming situations in your life as opportunities to make conscious, concise decisions. Staying stuck in indecision is paralysis caused by the ego's mind games. Don't let uncertainty keep your mind and body static. Instead, focus clearly on what you want by moving your attention away from what no longer aligns with you. If a wave of overwhelm rushes over you, stop, pause, direct your attention to your higher self, and communicate with your soul. Let your true self be your compass. When you are clear within yourself, you can relax into the natural rhythms of life and move forward with ease and joy.

I make decisions easily and am clear about what is most important to me. I choose to align to the choices that are advised by my higher self for optimum health and happiness.

RESTFUL RITUAL

Make an easy decision tonight by setting out your clothes for a smoother morning tomorrow.

I REST SO THIS CAN PASS.

If you are going through a difficult time in your life, your instinct may be to try to get past it as quickly as you can. The best thing you can do, however, is stop trying so hard to fix, solve, or move past the difficult time; instead, surrender deeply into it. Give yourself more gentleness by accepting what is; don't force the outcome. Be fully present in the uncomfortable aspects of your experience. The same way seeds lie dormant in winter, you can bloom from the hard times of your life with the right conditions. Give yourself proper care and know you will resurface soon, blooming bright with new life.

I grow from the ground up, rising higher with each passing season. I reach for the sky and let the light of my soul illuminate my path.

RESTFUL RITUAL

Give yourself a break by considering a different viewpoint tonight. Sit next to a houseplant and write a poem or a letter from the plant's perspective. What wisdom and advice does the plant have for you?

I AM AN EMOTIONAL ALCHEMIST.

Any internal conflict you feel could contradict beliefs at odds with each other. If you feel you're doing the inner work yet still feel criticism (from yourself or others), it could be because the emotional energy stored in your body has not been fully addressed. Our bodies hold the energy of past experiences, and if you've gone through a traumatic situation, it could feel unsafe to explore it. Energetic therapies like somatic healing can support you on your healing journey. Seek out routines and rituals that explore your body's painful experiences in a nurturing manner. Alchemize emotional healing in your body with intention and compassion.

I explore the depths of emotions in my body, acknowledging those that are trapped and unknown. I bravely explore my inner world to find healing and peace.

RESTFUL RITUAL

Try this somatic standing awareness stretch before bed: Stand with your feet rooted on the floor, and sway your body gently back and forth. Scan your body from top to bottom, observing how your muscles feel when you focus attention on them.

Blessings are always coming my way.

What do you consider successful and how do you measure progress? So often, we look outside of ourselves at the achievements of others (in our community, culture, even globally), then use these criteria to validate (or invalidate) ourselves. This validation can feel like forward movement, but the truth is, craving attention is driven by our ego, not our true self; nor is it any true indication of success. True progress is what happens on the *inside* and manifests outward—life's greatest blessing. Look inward to see how far you've come—how much you show up for yourself and how this blesses the world.

I am a great person and I am already blessed.
I feel good about my choices, knowing
that I live from the inside out, doing what
feels right to my true self.

Restful Ritual

Tonight, go to one of your favorite places in your home and sit with yourself in silence. List in your head or journal all the blessings you are grateful for and look forward to receiving.

I SHED THE LAYERS OF STRESS AND DECOMPRESS.

You want to be loved for who you are at your core. Unfortunately, even when you bravely show the deeper aspects of yourself, you may feel misunderstood and unappreciated; this could cause you to withdraw or react negatively, closing yourself off from the deep connections you crave.

It's hard for others to be there for you when there are aspects of yourself that you have not been there for—parts of you that you don't understand or appreciate. Tonight is an opportunity to honor and value your individuality. Be loyal to yourself by honoring your true self. The connection, meaning, and honesty you long for in your relationships are precious gifts you must first give to yourself.

I promise that I will never betray or
abandon myself—I am my greatest ally.
I am loyal and respectful to me,
and my relationships follow suit.

RESTFUL RITUAL

Turn your evening face-cleansing routine into a mini spa-like facial. Wash away the stress in circular, slow motions, taking this time to be loyal and honoring to yourself.

I SHOW RESPECT TO OTHERS BY TRUSTING THEIR AUTONOMY.

We've all had moments where we think we know what's best for others, but even with pure intentions, we still cross a boundary. Trust others by showing respect for their autonomy. Setting boundaries is about self-care and recognizing how much we can tolerate at any given time. If someone has set a boundary with you and you feel rejected, take a step back, realize this is a boundary violation and the potential start of a unhealthier cycle that could cause even more hurt and disappointment. Self-reflect on why you feel rejected or abandoned. See the lessons for you so you can heal and feel less triggered; this violation is often about you, and an apology is needed to repair the connection. To foster healthy relationships with others, you must first address the shaky boundaries within your own self.

I let go of my need to control any outcome or person and focus on myself. I drop deeper into the moment, honoring my internal landscape and its needs.

RESTFUL RITUAL

Set some boundaries for yourself by scheduling stress-free "me" time tonight. Remove any distractions and free your mind of worry. Listen to a calming meditation app or sounds of nature.

I RESPOND AS A LEADER IN DIFFICULT SITUATIONS.

Consider the qualities of an outstanding leader: a leader inspires, motivates, and adjusts to ever-shifting daily demands. Become the leader of your own life. Respond more swiftly, observing how different dynamics require you to pivot when needed. Embrace new opportunities and challenges, especially in regard to your own operating system. Your mind is like a computer running software (your thoughts and beliefs), but you may be operating on an outdated version. It's time to update and align with the latest version of you. Make sure you are not trying to solve new problems with old thinking. Tonight, fall asleep knowing that you are the leader in your own life.

I am a leader in my own life, and I stand proud in difficult situations. I adjust to the circumstances that I am living in and lead the path forward with love.

RESTFUL RITUAL

In your journal tonight, brainstorm some ideas on how you and others can solve a problem you're facing together.

I FIND CALM AND SERENITY BY CONNECTING TO MY HEART SPACE.

You are not at the mercy of everything that is happening to and around you. Call in calm by intentionally focusing on serenity. Bring your mental, physical, and emotional bodies into full alignment by accessing your heart's intuitive guidance. Take some time to nourish your heart by listening to its guidance and honoring what it needs, for your spiritual self (your soul) resides in your heart space. If you've been overwhelmed and stressed out, expand deeper into your heart chakra; it will lead you to serenity through the language of your soul.

I listen to my heart space to access calm and serenity. I release heavy thoughts to the care of its wisdom, and recognize its powerful guidance.

RESTFUL RITUAL

Before bed tonight, activate and rebalance your heart chakra. Take your right hand and hover it over your heart. Move your hand counterclockwise five times—this process recalibrates the energy. Then do the same rotation clockwise for five rotations—this helps to balance and stabilize your chakras.

I FEEL SO I CAN HEAL.

If you've recently received a distressing diagnosis, or if you're suffering from another imbalance or ailment, this is not the time for blame or negativity. Instead, begin to heal aspects of this condition by identifying the emotion that is tied to it. For example, if you've been suffering from migraines, your hurting head makes it hard for you to see. Ask yourself, *What have I been afraid to see in life?* Maybe your brain is exhausted from overthinking and needs time to rest. There's an emotion tied to your beliefs and ailments. Once you identify the emotion, you begin the journey to healing.

I recognize the connection between my body and my brain and the ways in which they communicate with one another to bring me into optimal balance. I support this relationship through the language of love and gratitude.

RESTFUL RITUAL

Prepare for bed by doing some gentle tai chi movements, connecting your inner world with your outer auric field and your head to your heart. (There are many short videos online if you've not tried it before.)

I RELEASE ALL OVERWHELM AND FIND SACREDNESS IN MY SILENCE.

In the digital age of social media, where information is blasted everywhere and oversharing is the norm, moving in silence can feel like a radical act of bravery. Keeping things to yourself is a powerful choice of self-care, however. When you keep your life's special moments sacred and private, you protect your own energy. Take some time to retract your energy and spend less effort being "seen" online; live your life more intentionally. Sometimes the best thing you can do is stay silent and under-share. Focusing on yourself and your loved ones is more important than trying to keep up with social media and its constantly changing algorithm. Get back to the divine source energy by reconnecting with yourself.

I free myself from overwhelm by living my life more privately. I release the need for outside validation, choosing to share because I care. My silence is safe and sacred.

RESTFUL RITUAL

Replace an evening of screen time with an evening of quality time with loved ones, and reflect on the experience in your journal before bed. How do you feel compared to nights spent in front of screens and online?

I AM IN PERFECT BALANCE. THIS IS WHERE I THRIVE.

Staying balanced in your life requires a constant check-in between disorder and order, confusion and calm, non-coherence and coherence. There is a set point in your life where balance can thrive; this is the median where creative potential exists. If you lean too heavily into your masculine energy—doing, achieving, and forcing—you'll be off-balance; and if you lean too heavily into your feminine energy—the parts of you that are passive and waiting—nothing will ever get done. Meet yourself in the middle; this is where stability and creative potential ignite.

I do not wait on my happiness or postpone my joy, nor do I rush into it. I am balanced and focus on the creative potential within.

RESTFUL RITUAL

Balance yourself with some gentle yoga poses before bed. Some good poses to do before bedtime are lotus position, downward dog, cow, cat, and child's pose.

I LET MY WALLS COME DOWN AND SHOW MY VULNERABILITY.

The walls set around your life are important, protecting you and providing boundaries to ensure that people respect your needs. But sometimes these walls are so high that they keep people out to an extreme. Are you pushing people away energetically because of past pain? If you've shared yourself with others in a vulnerable way and it was not reciprocated, it doesn't mean that you are unlovable. You gave a beautiful gift—you shared the real you. Let your walls down and focus on showing more of your true self to those who deserve to know you.

I am vulnerable with the people I care about and those who are close to me; I keep my best interests at heart. This is a gift to myself and them.

RESTFUL RITUAL

Focus on removing any masks you wear in your life by putting on a face mask before bed. Take the time to enjoy the process of taking or washing it off and feeling refreshed.

I AM THANKFUL FOR MY BEAUTIFUL BODY.

When is the last time you thanked your body for always being there for you? It is working for you and listening to your thoughts all the time. If you're sending your body negative thoughts, it's hearing that and responding. Your body is doing the best that it can to optimize itself in every moment. But when you're fighting against yourself, it's extra hard to give yourself time to really celebrate and honor your own body with rest and rejuvenation. Connect more deeply to your body and really appreciate it. Make it a point to regularly thank it, and thank yourself for loving it in return.

My body is a vehicle that holds my heart and head, where logic and love can exist at the same time. I celebrate my body and all that it's done and continues to do for me.

RESTFUL RITUAL

When you lie down on your bed tonight, sink into the mattress and let your body sink into and feel the softness of the blankets. Appreciate your body and give yourself a big hug.

I AM INHERENTLY WORTHY.

When you don't need validation from anyone else, you are the strongest force to be reckoned with. You are empowered by the knowledge of how amazing you already are—stronger than those who dwell in their insecurities and fear. Knowing your worth means you know who you are and what you stand for; you do not doubt yourself because you trust your own inner authority. You are strong within, and this is the greatest force in the world! You realize that you don't need to belong, to fit in—you are enough on your own.

I belong to myself and believe in my inner authority. I show up fully as myself in the world and live without fear, because I know I am inherently worthy.

RESTFUL RITUAL

In your journal tonight, think about one of your strengths and about someone who disrespects this strength. Write down the boundary you'd like to set and mentally convey it to them.

I INFUSE LOVE INTO THE PAIN OF MY PAST.

A lot of pain has been cast on you by other people, some with malicious intent and others unknowingly, and both by the wreckage of the unhealed parts of themselves; some may have left you feeling alone and misunderstood. But the more you heal and connect with your true self, the more you realize that you are composed of love, and the betrayals of the past are not a reflection of you. Part of healing is seeing things in a new light. Infuse more love into the pain of your past by recognizing that everyone operates from their own level of self-love and consciousness at any given time. You can infuse any hurtful memories with more love for yourself and allow yourself to move on.

I release my need for resolution or closure.
I send prayers to those who have harmed me,
and I let go with love and forgiveness.
I free myself of past pain.

RESTFUL RITUAL

As you fall asleep, remember that everyone deserves love. Can you send people who may have hurt you in the past a little bit of love? If it feels difficult to do at this time, start by sending your past self more love and forgiveness.

I CHOOSE TO SEE THE POSITIVE IN NEGATIVE SITUATIONS.

Some situations cause so much destruction that we feel like everything is crumbling around us. When you find yourself in this type of experience of life, where nothing you do seems to work or fix the situation and you feel negative and out of control, it's an opportunity to see the positive within the experience. There's always a light at the end of the tunnel. If you are in a tunnel right now, this is your opportunity to look for the light and activate positive experiences, even when you are drowning in the dark. If you feel that you are lost in the shadows, turn on your own inner light to find the solution.

I am a beacon of hope and love in a dark world. I turn on the light of positivity in me to guide myself and others.

RESTFUL RITUAL

Before bed, welcome the positive by imagining that you are a lighthouse shining your warm and loving light out into the world, onto everybody and everything.

I PROTECT MY ENERGY BY SAYING NO.

As you wind down tonight, protect your energy by reclaiming your personal space. Look at what you can say no to. Perhaps you can say no to doing the laundry, cleaning up after dinner, a last-minute invite from friends, or putting away the dishes. If you don't live alone, consider telling those around you that you need some self-care time, then go take care of *you*. Communicating your needs allows you to feel more empowered and supported. Focusing on your own well-being is in loving service to you, helping you rest your body, relax your mind, and feel more at ease.

I focus on self-care by communicating with those around me about my needs. I choose to say no when appropriate so that I can say yes to myself.

RESTFUL RITUAL

As you drift off to dreamland, identify a time you said no, perhaps when others wanted you to say yes. Revel in how good it feels to do things that align with your true self.

I BRAVELY CHANNEL MY EXPERIENCES TO HELP OTHERS HEAL.

What you go through helps you grow, and there are other people who are going through what you have just healed from. Additionally, there are some who go through these hard periods and look at others who are doing better with judgment, anger, and resentment. Remember that what we put out into the world, even in the forms of thought, we get back. No matter what is happening in your life, always turn to gratitude, grace, and a wish for the good will of all. Demonstrate this by helping others after you've healed. Ask yourself, *How can my personal experience help to uplift and support someone else?*

I help others through my awareness and understanding of my journey. I am called from a place of genuine support and care to assist them through difficult times.

RESTFUL RITUAL

Before bed write down the ways you could share the experiences you've overcome to benefit others. Maybe it involves joining a community group or starting an online program, anything that relates to what you've healed from can help as you share your experience and educational tips.

I TRANSCEND BEYOND MY LIMITING BELIEFS.

Whether it's a person, a belief system, cultural conditioning, political doctrine, or fear itself, deception casts a shadow over the light. If you feel yourself stuck in darkness, look at the beliefs you've been holding; maybe you have a mindset that no one can be trusted or that you are unlovable. Imagine yourself having a nightmare in a lucid state: you have the power to change directions and redirect the storyline by looking at the beliefs that are limiting you. Do you believe that you're not good enough for some desired result? To get new outcomes in life, we must transcend our limiting beliefs and release the fears driving our actions. Believe and know that you are worthy of more.

I do not allow fear to attach to and weigh down my experience of life. I transcend fear by choosing to live in light and love.

RESTFUL RITUAL

Shed the worries of the day by breathing deeply into your diaphragm and releasing tension as you exhale. This practice releases endorphins to calm your nervous system and invite rest.

I RELEASE MY INNER TURMOIL AND TRUST MY INSTINCTS.

Think about when you were younger and you had your whole life ahead of you: it was an era of excitement and wonder—you were carefree! But where did all that excitement go? You can combat the heavy energy of adult life and responsibilities by reclaiming this excitement in your life now. What dreams and goals did you have when you were a child? What kind of person did you want to be? You can still be that person by trusting your instincts and releasing self-doubt. Break free from the need for others' approval and the demands of daily life. Reconnect with your inner child to feel more balanced, aligned, and guided by your heart's deepest desires.

I am in tune with my internal compass. I reach for excitement, especially when I feel inner angst, because feeling is always healing.

RESTFUL RITUAL

Release your extra energy before bed. Pick one of your favorite songs from high school and dance it out. Shake your body and release the kinks between you and the flow of good vibe previously blocked from within.

I AM NOT MY PAST.
I KNOW MY INNER TRUTH.

The next time you feel like you have to defend yourself, check in first by asking yourself, *How am I feeling? Why do I feel defensive?* Insecurities from the past have a habit of playing out in the present, and there could be a past hurt, betrayal, or inconsistency raising its head in this situation; you may be defending yourself from a wounded memory imprint and not from the current reality. When this happens, step back and realize that you don't need to defend yourself. Redirect your energy toward healing what's coming up from the past. Those who live in the present—their truth—live an easier, happier life.

I do not need to defend myself for there's nothing to prove. I heal my past to better my current reality. I choose to live in my truth and feel good now.

RESTFUL RITUAL
Tonight, lighten your mood and invite curiosity of your inner child by reading from a book in a genre you have never read before but have always wanted to.

My relationships are nurturing and supportive.

Have you ever been around a group of people (coworkers, friends, or family) and felt royally misunderstood after you said something? Sometimes the people closest to us can make us feel the most unseen, even if they don't mean to. Other times, people aren't so kind, and they push back. Sharing your feelings with them and having respectful communication is important. Surround yourself with people who show up for you and honor how amazing you are. Reflect on your social sphere: Do you have reciprocal friendships and supportive circles? Shift away from people who bring you down or suck your energy. Focus on creating more genuine connections with loving people.

In my life, I choose people who see my value, for I know my worth. I am open to receiving abundant support in the form of rewarding, genuine, honest, and sincere friendships.

Restful Ritual

Soften your sleep tonight through the warmth of connection. Snuggle close with a loved one or a pet, or call someone who always makes you feel good.

THE LIGHT OF THE MOON ILLUMINATES WHAT HOLDS ME BACK.

The light and dark sides of the moon often symbolize the light and shadow sides of the self. You can use the energy of the moon's light to illuminate your inner world and its shadows. For example, you may be working hard to start your own business, doing your due diligence on all the key action steps, yet something holds back your success. Is there an ingrained belief that you can't make money doing what you love or that you are unworthy of achieving your heart's desires? This contrast is making things harder than they need to be. Invite more light into your inner world to transmute these fears into victories.

The moonlight cleanses lowering vibrations, thoughts, and fears in my life. I am connected to my true self and my purpose. I have all I need to succeed.

RESTFUL RITUAL

Tonight, do a moon meditation where you call in the moon's energy to wash away uncertainty and fear. Invite the moon's light to illuminate all that has been holding you back.

149

ALL IS THE WAY IT IS SUPPOSED TO BE.

We live in a world that puts a lot of pressure on us to be more than we are or have more than we do. It can feel like you're never getting ahead—yet another illusion that keeps you from realizing how magnificent you already are. You don't need material possessions to show the world how great you are or how successful you can be, nor do you need to prove anything to anyone. Free yourself from any ego-based expectations or worries, for your status and reputation mean nothing if you aren't comfortable with yourself. Fall in love with your own life exactly the way it is.

I am right where I need to be—all is in right order. I am not driven by ego needs or empty desires. I choose my path with truth and love.

RESTFUL RITUAL

Nothing clears internal spaces better than clearing external ones! Tonight, before bed, treat yourself to just that by decluttering a space that gets neglected, such as your bathroom cabinets and drawers.

My priorities shift when I am kind to myself.

When was the last time you prioritized self-love and self-care? Taking time for you is not just about physical care, such as bubble baths or massages; it is also about how you talk to yourself about yourself. Is your inner voice kind or is it derogatory? Are you constantly telling yourself you're not good enough, not doing a good job, not where you should be in life, not pretty enough, not smart enough, etc.? Well, enough is enough! It's time to turn that inner critic into a kind and compassionate friend. When you're kind to yourself, everything else in your life falls into alignment and becomes easier.

I speak kindly to myself—I am my own best friend. I know that I matter, and I know that I'm important. The way that I speak to myself is a reflection of this.

Restful Ritual

Write down ten things that you enjoy about yourself in your journal, and read them out loud to yourself before you go to sleep.

The world I see is not as it is but as I am.

Everyone on the planet has unique opinions and personal history that make up their worldviews. Is there a part of you that believes other people should see things the way you do? Or perhaps you've been frustrated because people don't. Everyone has their own perspectives and experiences. In light of this rich diversity, connecting with others should be exciting! Share your views, and listen to others with curiosity. Rest comfortably in your own knowing—you don't need other people to see things the same way to be confident in connecting.

I accept others for who they are and let them be. I see myself surrounded by people of like mind and heart when I show the real me.

Restful Ritual

Tonight, choose a person you've been in conflict with and focus on putting yourself in their shoes. Set the intention to have a lucid dream to better understand and connect peacefully with this person, so you may resolve your conflict amicably in real life.

Anxious thoughts
are not my truth.

When anxious thoughts arrive, you don't have to buy into them or make them part of your reality. See your thoughts as driftwood passing by in a river rather than a logjam interrupting the flow of your life. Driftwood moves along gracefully, shifting through the water. When you meditate, you can start to take ownership of your thoughts and keep them moving too. Let them pass by like driftwood. If an anxious thought comes in, acknowledge it for what it is: it is not your reality, nor is it your truth. Focus on what you know is true and real, and let the rest pass by.

Fear and worry are not my reality—I do not dwell in them. I put energy and focus on what I can control and what I can do, and send the rest away with love.

Restful Ritual

Fall asleep to the sounds of ocean waves tonight. (You can search online for recordings and videos, or use a meditation app. Or if you are lucky enough to live by the sea, open the window.)

I CHOOSE TO BE CONSCIOUS OF MY BLIND SPOTS.

When we ignore our own insecurities, fears, and shadows, we ignore important parts of ourselves. These blind spots are teachers, not adversaries. We might even blame other people, but the situation is not their fault. To eliminate the dark areas, we must first take accountability. Tonight is an opportunity to go inward and see *your* role in the situations causing you stress. Have you been participating as a victim or a victor? Take control of your autonomy and your strengths! Both are more than enough to see you through.

I show up with respect for others and accountability for my actions. I know that every difficult experience is an opportunity to learn and grow.

RESTFUL RITUAL

Realign your perspective by activating all your senses before bed. Take a deep breath in, and as you release it, identify five things in your surroundings that you can *see*, then (after breathing in again) four things that you can *hear*, then three things that you can *touch*, then two things you can *smell*, then one thing you can *taste*.

I FILL UP MY CUP WITH SELF-LOVE AND IT BALANCES ME.

Your level of self-love and self-awareness dictate your ability to show up for others. When you go on a personal growth journey, but others around you are not ascending, it can cause conflict. Others may react in ways that seem harmful. The reality is, when you grow, not everyone around you will go in the same direction, and this can hurt emotionally. But don't sacrifice your healing—hold up the energetic mirror. The outside world is a reflection of our internal state. Commit to meeting these needs within yourself first. For example, if you don't feel understood in a relationship, ask yourself what part of yourself you have ignored. Commit to approaching and honoring your whole self more through all stages of your healing and personal growth journey.

I take the necessary time to focus on me, nurturing my mind, body, and spirit. When I do this, I think better, I feel better, and I do better. I live from a place of wholeness.

RESTFUL RITUAL

Prepare for bedtime with a stress-busting adaptogen latte: in your favorite mug or teacup, mix one cup of hot water or your favorite milk with one to two teaspoons of cocoa and one teaspoon of ashwagandha,[32] or reishi (all stress-fighting herbs), and sweeten to taste. Sip in bliss and enjoy.

I ADD GREAT VALUE AND MAKE A DIFFERENCE IN THE WORLD.

What keeps you up at night? Where is your heart feeling called to support and lead? Focus on a single cause that is important to you. So many different areas in the world could benefit from your efforts, but you have a special focus and passion motivating you and it is time to honor it. When you tap into this unique calling, you're able to make more of a difference. Return to your heart's bidding, helping where and when you can.

I release the need to be everything to everyone—I cannot give my attention to all needs on the planet. I surround myself with positive energy and focus on how I can help in my own way.

RESTFUL RITUAL

Tonight, identify a cause that is important to you and consider how you can best serve it. How can you give more of your time, money, energy, or support? Make a plan to help this week, where and when you can.

I AM WILLING TO SEE AND EMBRACE THE TRUTH OF MYSELF. I AM HEALTHY, HAPPY, AND WHOLE.

When life gets to be too much, it's easy to turn to unhealthy crutches: addictions, negative thought patterns, vices—all the quick go-tos of relief that could cause more harm in the long run. Your true self doesn't need these to be happy. If you're returning to old habits and wish to stop, practice self-compassion (the related shame and blame is more detrimental than the actual activity). Start by being aware of your inner voice—what you are telling yourself about the situation? Instead of saying, *I am a horrible person and will never be free of this*, you could say this: *For today, I am doing the best I can, and I can do even better tomorrow. I am willing to see and embrace the truth of myself, healthy, happy, and whole.*

I disengage from harmful activities and habits. I am kind to and patient with myself as I step back into my whole, happy self.

RESTFUL RITUAL

Before bed, journal about a harmful habit that you'd like to replace with a healthier habit. Make a plan to start implementing the change this week. Remember it just takes one step, one day at a time, to make positive change.

I CHOOSE TO RELEASE MY ANGER AND WORRIES.

Anger is a valuable emotion, setting you free from feeling sad or frustrated. Yet anger is a destructive emotion too, when utilized irresponsibly. Many of us are taught to not feel angry, and we can become people pleasers to avoid the sensations of being angry. This emotion is important for you to process, however; it's guiding you to see what is important to you and to stand up for yourself. Often, anger arises when a boundary has been violated. If you have a situation where you feel angry, recognize this as an opportunity to speak up and share your truth.

My anger shows me what I care about—
where my boundaries are and when to protect
them. By honoring myself, I release the
anger and use my voice to stand up
for what matters most to me.

RESTFUL RITUAL

If you have pent-up energy tonight, release it in a healthy way: pop in your headphones and dance it out. Feel angry? Play a song with extra expressive lyrics and add air punches and kicks, or take it out on your pillow.

This is temporary, and I am strong enough to handle it.

Everything in front of you is also on its way out—what's coming is always going—and sooner or later, you will be done with it. (As the saying goes, "This, too, shall pass.") Do you want to perpetuate the stress in this situation or do you want to remove yourself from adding to it? You have the power to declare, "Access denied! I am not available to this experience anymore." Whatever is causing you angst, release the stress by reclaiming your power and deciding how much of your energy you're going to give it. Focus your attention, time, and energy on what truly supports and uplifts you.

What I'm going through is temporary and is not going to take me down with it. I remove myself from anything that is not in alignment by declaring my power is my peace, no matter what.

Restful Ritual

Tonight, reflect on a time in your life when you overcame something that was incredibly challenging. Identify and celebrate the skills and strength that you used to make it through.

I RID MYSELF OF ALL TOXICITY AND PRIORITIZE ME.

When was the last time you felt whole and healthy? We all have layers of toxicity in our lives that need to be cleansed regularly. Just like when you do a detox or fast to reset your body, you can do a life clean-up by clearing out clutter beyond this. Toxicity builds up in the form of negativity, low-level vibrational habits, environmental toxins, chemicals in foods, and the bad behaviors of unhealed people in our lives. When you go on a healing journey, you raise your vibration and your standards. You no longer feel good in low-vibration situations, and unhealthy habits naturally fall away. Prioritize your health by clearing away toxicity, and enjoy how your life improves.

My mental, physical, and energetic health are connected, and what I surround myself with matters. I rid myself of toxicity and clutter to elevate my well-being.

RESTFUL RITUAL

Refresh and cleanse the air quality of your sleeping space by investing in an air purifier for your bedroom or opening a window to bring in fresh air.

I INVITE POSITIVE ENERGY TO FLOW THROUGH MY BODY.

If you want anything in your life, it's important to invite it in. Sometimes we don't realize we are blocking our own desires by focusing on the lack. Turn your attention away from the deficit by inviting positive energy to flood through your body with good-feeling sensations—this is a practice you can cultivate every evening. And as you start to feel better within your body, you become a manifesting magnet for all the things that you seek. Focus your attention on the abundant energy of love and possibilities to expand into a higher vibration of gratitude and attract the things that you wish for.

I attune to the abundance all around and within me. I am a magnificent creator when I align with positive energy and flow.

RESTFUL RITUAL

Lie down in your bed before you go to sleep, grab a crystal (black tourmaline if you have one—it helps remove negativity), and place on your heart. Invite positive energy to flow through your entire body, like a wave energetically vibrating through every cell.

As I welcome sleep, I celebrate my good deeds.

You are a good person, and you've spent time, money, and energy to get to the state you are in right now. Think about all the things you did just today that actually took a lot of time and effort to do and that have likely gone unnoticed. Tonight, take a moment to really celebrate all that you're doing for yourself and your loved ones. Welcome your sleep as a respite you've wholeheartedly earned, and you'll sleep well knowing that you had a good day. Focus on the good deeds that ripple through the world because of you being wonderful you.

I focus on all that is well. When I reflect upon the goodness of each day, I rest peacefully through the night.

Restful Ritual

As you get settled into bed, take a *good-day* inventory. Mentally map out all the positive things that happened today as you drift off to sleep.

I HEAL MY MIND WITH NURTURING THOUGHTS AND ACTIVITIES.

Healing is a process, and it's not one-size-fits-all; some modalities that work for others may not work for you. If you're on a journey to find your best healing path, pay attention to what is aligned with and uplifting to you, and create a routine that honors these tools and rituals. For example, if you love water, add more water therapy to your daily routine (a hot bath, cold plunge, or swimming); if you love nature and feel calmed by trees, make sure you get into nature every day, and get more real houseplants. Fill your mind with nurturing thoughts that are connected to feeling well, as this is part of your healing journey—the path to your optimal well-being.

I focus on body balance, doing activities each day that bring harmony and peace. I honor what is important to me by structuring my life around rituals and routines that make me feel good.

RESTFUL RITUAL

Tonight, identify a nurturing activity that you absolutely love. Plan at least one day this week to go and do this activity.

163

I BECOME SLEEPIER WITH EACH BREATH I TAKE.

Every breath you take is an opportunity to invite a deeper life force into your vessel. Imagine that breathing is a special ceremony dedicated to you—a ceremony honoring you as a gift of continued life. Consciously fill your lungs with air as you bring more energetic flow and higher vibrations to your life. Oxygen is medicine, so focus on bringing more of it into your body, giving thanks for how it balances and regulates your system. Fall deeper into sleep as your body relaxes into the ceremony of you.

As I breathe consciously into my vessel, I see how important I truly am. Sleep is a ritual that I honor each day by breathing deeper into the night.

RESTFUL RITUAL

Do a breath exercise before bed: Inhale slowly through your nose and count to five in your head, filling your lungs with more air with each number. Hold for five seconds, then slowly exhale gently through your mouth, pushing all the oxygen softly out of your lungs. Repeat as needed until you drift off to sleep.

I AM SAFE AND SECURE RIGHT NOW.

Many people suffer from PTSD or CPTSD, especially veterans. Whether you've been in the service or are simply fighting your own past trauma, moving from debilitating experiences to safety can feel impossible to navigate. One way to transition more smoothly is to do a ritual cleansing. Ancient civilizations, such as Rome, used to consider war a ritual and understood the need for returning war heroes to purify themselves before coming back into society. Ceremonies such as bathing them to "purge them of the corruption of war" were essential.[33] You can also *purge* any heaviness form your day before bed by ritualizing your healing to improve your sleep each night.

I cleanse myself and feel secure by releasing past stories, stress, and pain. I recognize that I am safe, here and now.

RESTFUL RITUAL

Before bed, take a steam shower. Add a few drops of bergamot or palo santo essential oil to the shower floor, and run the hot water long enough to create a steady flow of steam. While in the shower, focus on releasing feelings of grief, hopelessness, and despair and taking in love, peace, and hope.

I GRACEFULLY MOVE PAST STUCK AND STATIC ENERGY.

No matter how hard you try, you cannot force an outcome; it may feel like you take two steps forward, then four steps back. Whether you can't seem to get on the same page with another person or you keep falling short of the goal you're trying to reach, feeling let down by life can take a toll. When life sucks the life out of you, it's time to regroup by focusing your energy elsewhere. It may be time to learn a new skill or improve a natural talent. Tap into your creativity to get energy moving again.

My skills are my tools to move through stuck energy. When I feel blocked, I take action by learning new things. I am never stuck when I am growing.

RESTFUL RITUAL

Tonight, take one of the burdens that have been stressing you out and imagine that you're putting it into a box and closing it; then hand it over to whatever higher power you identify with, saying, "I release you into the light."

I BREAK OUT OF PATTERNS THAT HOLD ME BACK.

It makes sense to move away from things that cause pain. Whether you've gone through a breakup, left a job, or dislike where you live, a change of scene can be helpful. There are times when you're not running toward but *away*, however. The problem? You can't run away from the things that live within you. Look at the stressors in your life and see if you've been running away from anything to try to make your life easier. When you run away by removing yourself physically or by energetically checking out, it's likely the stressful situations will repeat themselves. Until you face your inner turmoil head-on, wherever you go, there you are.

I am open to seeing things differently and shifting when necessary. My choices are effortless when I am in tune with myself. I am always right where I need to be.

RESTFUL RITUAL

Put on your cozy slippers, and walk around your bedroom. Ask yourself, *Am I running toward what I want or running away from myself?* Reflect on the answers you receive.

I FACE MY SHADOW TO BETTER UNDERSTAND MY LIGHT.

Do you have anyone in your life with whom you're unable to be your true self? If this person only likes it when you are a certain way, you are already hiding parts of yourself that you're afraid they won't accept or love. Use this as an invitation to recognize the beautiful, expansive world inside you. All your feelings and understandings about life are valid—light and dark, happiness and sadness, fear and love—and they can coexist; one isn't more important than the other. When you show up as your true self, it gives others the opportunity to meet you with the same love and respect.

I acknowledge the feelings that I wish to hide from the world by processing them. I feel best when I show up for others by first showing up for myself. I honor my shadow and my light.

RESTFUL RITUAL

Since your bed holds energy like everything else in your home, try cleansing its energy by removing all clutter and unnecessary items from under and around it. You can also refresh the energy by washing the sheets and changing out the pillowcases and or blankets.

I PUT MY EGO ASIDE IN THIS MOMENT.

Your ego lives in your mind—it's the part of you that *thinks* rather than *feels*. But your thoughts are not always real; they are observations. The ego wants you to believe that every thought you have is important, and this can cause harm, especially when the thoughts are more painful than the actual circumstances themselves. For this moment, rest your weary mind and put your thoughts aside. Try to empty your mind and be present. There is nothing to achieve, do, or be—you don't have to figure anything out. Release all expectations, free your mind of thoughts, and for this moment, just be.

I have nothing else to focus on except this moment, right here and now. My overwhelming thoughts dissipate, and all that is left is authentic.

RESTFUL RITUAL

Warmth invites comfort and relaxation before bed. Place a heated wrap on your neck or forehead to start the process, perhaps adding a drop or two of lavender oil to enhance the experience.

169

I LOVE AND APPRECIATE MYSELF— I DID WELL TODAY.

When is the last time that you said *I love you* to yourself? How often do you actually look in the mirror and say kind things about beautiful, one-of-a-kind *you*? Are you making it through your day and going into the night without ever acknowledging yourself? Make tonight a celebration of all that you are and all that you do for yourself and those around you. Honor and respect your goodness—you did well today; you *really* did! Take this moment to celebrate, honor, and appreciate you. Accept yourself consciously and fully, inside and out.

*I embrace myself with overflowing love.
I allow myself to be fully present in my life's
journey by showing up and acknowledging
how good and worthy I am. All is well when
I accept and love myself dearly.*

RESTFUL RITUAL

Before you go to bed, look into your eyes in a mirror, and tell yourself three ways you love and appreciate yourself.

I EMBODY THE LOVE THAT IS ME.

How much of your time do you spend picking apart, analyzing, or judging yourself? We are often our own worst critic, saying things to ourselves that aren't kind, let alone true. When you believe these thoughts about yourself, it's harder to feel good. Love who you are, as love created you: *love* is what you are made of. Tonight is a reminder that anytime you feel overwhelmed by negative thoughts, you can return to your center—to the source of love that created you. Feel the love that is around and inside of you *always*.

The love that I have for myself is the truth,
for I was created in love. I live, breathe, and
act from love. I am love, through and through.

RESTFUL RITUAL

Before bed, reconnect with yourself by placing both hands on your heart. Imagine your breath is flowing in and out of this area. Breathe a little deeper and slower than you normally would, inhaling for five counts and exhaling for five counts. Repeat this pattern until you fall asleep.

I AM A WARRIOR, NOT A WORRIER.

You have warrior energy that vibrates in every cell of your body—we all do. It's a universal life force, and you get to tap into this energy to make the most of your life in the way that you see fit. If worries get in the way of you slaying the day, however, this force can feel burdensome. You are brave and strong, and you will never be handed anything that you were not meant to excel through and overcome. Tonight, discover the warrior energy inside of you, like a phoenix rising from the ashes. Boldly move forward, proud and resilient.

I let go of worry to rise into the present moment and the warrior that I am. Strength, resilience, and bravery are my birthright.

RESTFUL RITUAL

Prepare for rest with an energy reset. Stand up and put your body in a power stance, like a superhero. Puff up your chest, and take up space by spreading your arms and legs wide. Feel empowerment and confidence flowing through your body.

My experiences shape me into who I am meant to be.

Look at your life through the lens of love: do you see that everything you've gone through has helped you become who you are? Every moment of your life is significant— there is a reason things happen the way they do. Everyone you've met has been on your path for a reason as well. There are villains and there are victors, and you can be either in your own life story. When you engage with life through this lens, it's easier to write the script as you want and redirect your story if things feel off. Grab your popcorn and enjoy the show!

Every experience I have helps me grow. My entire life is an amazing gift of adventure that I craft into who I am today.

Restful Ritual

Do some visualization before bed, imagining your life as a movie and you as the star. What kind of movie have you been living, and what experiences do you want to produce moving forward?

There is power and growth in forgiveness.

People can only show up with the amount of self-love and inner work that they have done on themselves. Sadly, it's impossible to ask someone else to see you or be there for you if they don't even know themselves. It's even harder to ask someone to show up for you when you're not showing up for yourself. This process is not about condemning yourself or blaming anyone; it's about honoring your role in your life, and how each person has come to you with a lesson or a blessing. Give yourself the same gift: learn the lessons and bless yourself with forgiveness. We can only forgive others by first forgiving ourselves.

My focus is on loving me. I choose compassion and forgive myself when necessary. I release the burden of pain by learning its lessons and moving on.

Restful Ritual

Grab your favorite worry stone to hold in your hand as you meditate or pray before bed. Focus on forgiving others by first forgiving yourself.

I HEAL IN DUE TIME. MY HEART IS WHOLE AND HEALTHY.

There is no expiration date on healing. When you open yourself to love, you open your inner world to vulnerability. If this sacred exchange is violated and you are let down by another, it makes opening up more difficult the next time. A broken heart is not really broken, however; it is a *full* heart that has expanded past its previous boundaries to reach new heights. The pain you feel from the loss is important to process, and it takes as long as it takes. Just remember that the reward of an expanded heart is expanded love in return.

My heart cracks wide open to expand, and I am healing. I embrace the feelings that come from my expanded heart, and I see that my heart is not broken. I show up with love because I am love, and this is never wrong.

RESTFUL RITUAL

Hum a self-love song to yourself as you fall asleep tonight, pouring all the love that you've been extending to others back into yourself.

I RID MYSELF OF NEGATIVE THOUGHTS TO PURIFY MY MIND AND BODY.

We all in suffer from exhaustion and information overload. Most of us are bombarded daily with an excess of information, usually online. Whether it is social media, world news on the television (and usually about what's going wrong), gossip from friends, or everyday conversations with family members, we are constantly being given new information. A lot of it is fear-based misinformation, created to evoke emotional responses and keep us trapped in a low-energy, low-vibrational state. Take some time to remove yourself from all distractions; time spent in nature is an excellent way to purify your mind and body. Clear your energy by realigning your external and internal boundaries to the things that matter most to you.

I clear my mind by focusing on positive intentions. The quality of my internal and external energy is important, and I cleanse mine daily.

RESTFUL RITUAL

Tonight, rid your home of dense, old energy. Smudge your space with birch bark or sage, or use some palo santo (for purification and energy cleansing) essential oil–infused spray.

I ILLUMINATE MY WORLD WITH COMPASSION.

When you are drowning in thoughts of negativity, pain, and worry, this lowers your vibration, keeping you from the light of your balanced, perfect center. Replace any negative thoughts with loving ones, filling your headspace with illumination and compassion whenever you need them. As you close your eyes and fall asleep tonight, bask in the energy of goodness, tuning out all negativity and harmful thinking. Feel uplifted and more connected to what is real by connecting to the buoyancy and lightness of positive thoughts and compassion.

I am a channel for light, and I embrace the love that I am. I remove dense energy and negativity from my thoughts and my perceptions. I choose not to worry and focus on the love that I have for myself and others instead. This love activates new possibilities and expansion.

RESTFUL RITUAL

Try wearing earplugs tonight when you sleep. It's a wonderful way to tune out noises that could disrupt your peaceful slumber.

My emotional, physical, and mental health are in harmony.

Your mental health is part of your overall health. How you feel each day is connected to your outlook and perspective on life. If you're feeling burdened and overwhelmed by everyday circumstances and demands, your mental health needs attention. Perhaps you feel unsatisfied, anxious, depressed, or lonely. Use your physical body to improve your mental well-being—all parts of you are connected. When your body moves, your mental and emotional body move too—focus on flushing out and processing any stuck energy. Enlist the motion of all these layers to yourself to maintain harmony and feel freer.

My mind, body, and spirit are one. My mental health is connected to my physical and spiritual health, and all contribute to my well-being. My mental health is strengthened by taking care of my body.

Restful Ritual

Before bed, put on a good song and move your body around your home in any manner that feels freeing. Practice the freedom of self-expression. As you listen to the emotive lyrics of the song, feel the vibrations in your body and open yourself to expressing the emotions that want to come through and be released.

I STAND UP FOR MYSELF WITH GRACE AND CONFIDENCE.

You have an important perspective to share with others; start speaking up on the things that matter most to you, and do so with grace and respect. You'll notice improvements in your life and your sleep when you do.

Take tonight to reflect upon your choices and your relationships: Do the people in your life see your value and honor you for who you truly are? Do you honor and respect yourself? If you don't stand up for yourself, no one else will. Have confidence, be bold, and use your voice to uphold your unique and inherent value.

I stand up for myself and my unique
perspective—no one else can do it for me.
I am confident in my worth and my beliefs;
they come from a place of love and respect.

RESTFUL RITUAL

Take a hot shower before bed to get your blood flowing away from your body's core. You can even use a few drops of eucalyptus essential oil for aromatherapy and recreate a spa-like experience. This drop in temperature and relaxing aroma can help you fall asleep faster.

MY DREAMS ARE VALID, AND I AM WORTHY OF ACTUALIZED ACHIEVEMENTS.

It's human nature to project the "likeable" parts of ourselves and hide the more authentic aspects; we all want to be loved and fit in. Unfortunately, the undertone of this behavior is fear of rejection and negative self-talk (called *imposter syndrome* when more deep-seated). If you feel like you suffer from self-doubt or have a sinking sensation you're going to be "found out," you could suffer from this malady. It's another form of feeling unworthy—a sneaky ego trick to keep us small in the face of our dreams. Instead of agonizing over your perceived flaws, be gentler with yourself. Realize that you can achieve great results when you believe in yourself. Embrace your unique, fun-loving self, and shoot for the stars!

I focus on the good, because I know I am worthy of my dreams and achievements. I transmute self-doubt into self-love.

RESTFUL RITUAL

Create an audio file on your smartphone of the mantra above and include a heartfelt message to yourself. Play it out loud before bed and anytime self-doubt creeps into your thoughts and goals.

I SLEEP BETTER WHEN I'M GROUNDED.

Walking around barefoot on the grass is a positive boost for your body. Research proves that grounding to the earth reduces body pain and inflammation, supports the body's stress response so it can stabilize faster, and improves your sleep state.[34] There are various grounding systems that can help you to connect to the earth while you sleep. When you touch the earth with your skin, you receive a charge of its energy and balance. Turn your bedroom into an Earth oasis, with plants, earth colors, and grounding stones and crystals to support a stronger sleep atmosphere.

My body is in harmony and I am in balance,
especially when I ground myself with Earth
energy. I fall asleep in this energy and let it
recharge me every night.

RESTFUL RITUAL

Grounding is crucial to a good night's sleep. Consider investing in some conductive (grounding) sheets, pillowcases, or blankets for your bed in the future; for tonight, bring a plant into your room and visualize "rooting" yourself to the earth through your bed.

I take responsibility for my home environment.

How often do you prioritize your environmental health? Removing toxicity from the home goes far beyond dusting furniture or clearing the cupboards of expired foods. Unprocessed emotions and heavy energies also occupy your home, and this increases when you share your space with someone else. If you feel like you're walking on eggshells or are cranky yourself, it's time to reconnect to love—first with yourself, then with your housemate. To heal the situation, focus on your self-care and life balance, adjust your environment to support this, and get adequate rest. Stay true to yourself and your optimal wellness. (And don't forget to forgive your housemate in the process!)

When my body needs to slow down, I honor its needs and prioritize rest. I create and maintain an environment that sustains my overall happiness and well-being.

Restful Ritual

Create an emotional place of safety and sanctuary in your bedroom. Pick an area that brings you comfort, and prepare the space with supportive things, like your favorite book, a cozy blanket, and candles.

My healing takes me to new places.

When you go on a personal growth journey, you travel to new, higher levels of awareness. One of the most important tools that you can access at any point along the way is your critical thinking. When you are open-minded and willing to look beyond what you already know to be true, your entire world shifts into expansive possibilities. This requires an ability to suspend your disbelief, temporarily holding off conflicting views and mental objections long enough to see if this new perspective feels right and resonant with your truth. And you will always know when it does from the freedom you feel within.

I live in a fluid cycle of healing, growth, and evolution. I stay open-minded and trust in my journey of expansion.

Restful Ritual

Head to bed a half hour earlier than you normally do; while you sit in bed, do hand yoga, stretching and relaxing your wrists and fingers.

My sleep is my freedom.

There is a freedom that comes with an excellent night's sleep—something we may not associate with a good night's rest. We probably think about how productive we can be in the day when we sleep well at night, but freedom is actually the feeling many of us are looking for when we sleep: freedom from body aches and pains, freedom from daily stresses, freedom from mental angst, and more.

Examine your rest routine to see if you are focusing on freedom or productivity. Freedom at night allows you to tap deeper into your dreams—into restorative REM sleep. Release the worries and mental frustrations of an over-stressed lifestyle by prioritizing the freedom of sleep.

I prioritize my sleep to make me feel
balanced on the inside and out—
the ultimate freedom.

Restful Ritual

Before going to bed or while in bed, use a heating or compression pad to free yourself of aches and pains and experience better sleep.

I INFUSE MY MORNING AND EVENING ROUTINES WITH GRATITUDE.

Focusing on what is wonderful in your life will help you feel good, especially when you prioritize positive thoughts as a daily and nightly intention. Consider infusing more positivity into your morning and evening routines: wake up with gratitude and go to bed with it too. Tonight is a reminder to focus on your evening routine to ensure that it is free of worry. Clear your mind of negativity by appreciating what is around you right now. As you focus more on the good, the stress and worry naturally slip away. Do this every day and night, and you'll start to feel better overall and especially as you drift off to sleep.

I prioritize gratitude and quality sleep as part of my morning and evening wellness routines. I tune in to positive thinking as my daily intent, and I feel better.

RESTFUL RITUAL

Tonight, look around your bedroom space and whisper to yourself "I am grateful for this" as you identify the things around you that you appreciate.

I SHARE MY LIFE STRUGGLES WITH HUMOR AND GRACE.

Undoubtedly, the most entertaining jokes are the ones we relate to on a collective level. There is nothing more relatable than sharing rock-bottom stories or situations of being stuck on the struggle bus. Let's face it: none of us can escape failure in life. Making people laugh with self-deprecating jokes can be a fun way to connect and break down walls; just be careful not to use your humor as a way of keeping people at bay. Sometimes when we make ourselves the butt of jokes, it's a trauma response—a way to protect our heart and vulnerability. Humor has its place and time, but always check in with yourself to see if your humor is bringing you closer to or further away from those around you.

I share my struggles through humor to bring people together. I allow myself to be vulnerable and honest, and I do so with self-respect and grace.

RESTFUL RITUAL

Allow extra time to unwind tonight, watching your favorite comedy movie, funny show, or online video before bed, or share a funny experience or story with a loved one.

I WELCOME THE UNIVERSE'S PLAN FOR ME.

Imagine going to a tarot card reader or psychic and asking, "When will I win the lottery?" or "When will I meet my soulmate?" Most likely, whatever they tell you won't feel good enough, because it isn't here now. Waiting for something you want is missing the point of living your life *today*; you cannot see the big picture or rush what is in store for you. You aren't supposed to know what's around the corner, and the universe doesn't want you to be on standby. Your life is meant to be lived, not controlled. Focus on living more intentionally and learning life's lessons, so you can be ready to receive what you desire in divine timing.

I release the expectation of how I think my life should be. I enjoy living intentionally while on my life's journey. I surrender all to divine timing.

RESTFUL RITUAL

Tonight, pull a card from the *Happy Bedtime Mantras Card Deck* or your favorite oracle or tarot card deck, and reflect on the reading in your journal.

I FOLLOW MY INTUITION OVER MY EMOTIONS.

Your emotions are important and valid, but they change often. It's important to recognize and honor them, but don't let them lead you. Instead, listen to your inner voice—the nudge; the gut feeling; the soft, wise awareness that lives within. For example, you could have emotions that say, "The person I just went on a date with is *so* fantastic. Wow! So much chemistry!" But your intuition is screaming, *Something is off!* And you realize that you felt a pit in your stomach the whole time. Was it butterflies or a warning? Deep down, you know the truth. Trust your intuition *always*. Emotions are fleeting.

I honor my emotions when they appear, but they are temporary—I let them pass. My intuition is my steadfast compass, guiding me to safety. I practice following it daily.

RESTFUL RITUAL

Before you turn out the light tonight, take a moment to understand yourself better through a personality test like the BigFive, Enneagram, or Human Design.

I AM NOT DEFINED BY WHAT OTHERS THINK OF ME.

When people misunderstand you or misrepresent you to others, you have several options: you can try to prove them wrong by speaking your truth, or you can let things lie and not defend yourself. While it may seem helpful to fight back, be sure your ego isn't leading the way; fighting back may cause more stress and anxiety than simply removing yourself from a no-win situation. In reality, you're stepping away to take the high road and protect your peace. Defend your precious energy by focusing on creating the life you want to live—one that is free of false information about you. The less you engage, the faster it goes away.

I am stronger than lies and manipulations—
I am free of what others think of me. I focus
my energy on creating a strong foundation of
truth and love in my life.

RESTFUL RITUAL

Free yourself of human entanglements by connecting with nature's energy before bed. Open a window to feel the night air or go outside and stargaze.

I AM IN CONTROL OF MY EMOTIONS AND IN BALANCE.

You probably have heard of testing for your IQ, but when is the last time you took an EQ test? Testing your EQ, or emotional intelligence quotient, indicates how you relate to and interact with others and yourself. Our relationships determine, in part, our quality of life. Think about how your emotions drive your actions: Are you a reactive person? Do you hold back your emotions out of fear? Do you believe showing vulnerability is a weakness? Having a healthy EQ means you're not reactive, you have a steady head on your shoulders, and you recover faster from negative emotions without getting derailed by daily dramas. Seek emotional balance to find overall balance.

I have accomplished amazing things in my life, and I appreciate all of me. It's all been worth it.

RESTFUL RITUAL

Prepare for rest by releasing a stuck emotion. Call upon your guides, angels, ancestors, or anyone else that you want to assist you. State aloud, "I am ready to release this emotion. I release it with ease."

THE MOON AMPLIFIES THE ENERGY IN MY LIFE.

In popular culture, the full moon is the scapegoat for most of the things that go bump in the night, from ghostly sightings to spikes in crime, to mood swings, to (you guessed it!) insomnia. If you've ever found yourself wide awake well past your bedtime, the full moon could be to blame, but this has more to do with light energy than dark. Sensitive souls and empathic people are usually more sensitive during the full moon, but anyone can balance their sleep cycle at any time by practicing compassion and kindness toward themselves and others. When you have trouble sleeping, simply draw your attention to your heart chakra by the light, loving energy of the moon.

The moon is a beacon of light illuminating
all that I need to see. I forgive and
release with compassion in my heart.
I am blessed beyond belief.

RESTFUL RITUAL

Certain food habits can help you relax and find better sleep. Pay attention to your diet. Before bed avoid sugars. Also, try to avoid gluten, which disturbs digestion.

I WALK THROUGH MY CONCERNS AND TAKE THE NEXT STEP.

Your concerns could be overpowering you and making it hard to move forward. Maybe you want to start a new project or get back into something that you used to love, but you find yourself procrastinating—a sign that you may be overthinking the outcome: *Will my endeavors work out? Will I be successful? Will I fail?* Perfectionism kicks in next, and you stay stuck. Consider for a moment that the concerns you have about the situation are actually *more* detrimental than the situation itself. Recognize, then release your concerns. Focus on taking one step at a time with clarity and confidence.

I acknowledge and release my concerns;
they don't hold me back. I'm inspired,
and I choose progress over procrastination
and perfectionism.

RESTFUL RITUAL

Try rhythmic chanting tonight, repeating the word *Om*. Concentrate on the sound, and feel the vibrations of the chant resonating within you. If your mind wanders, simply bring your focus back to the chant.

I LOVE DEEPLY AS A GIFT TO MYSELF AND THE WORLD.

Disappointments in love are a part of life—things don't always turn out the way you expected. It is essential to the human experience to give love as a gift, but it is mostly a gift to yourself. Showing up fully in your human expression—to give it all that you have—is beautiful and pure; loving is never wrong. And we have two choices when love doesn't turn out the way we had hoped: acceptance or anger. If someone has betrayed you or you're going through a breakup or divorce, love is still there for you in your own heart—your love for yourself will get you through. Open yourself to this love, and be an example of peace, even through the pain.

Love is the elixir—my medicine of choice.
I show up fully when I love myself fully.

RESTFUL RITUAL

Before bed, take out your journal or some pretty stationery, and write a love letter to yourself.

I MAKE THE REST OF MY LIFE THE BEST OF MY LIFE.

When is the last time you looked in the mirror and thought, *Wow, I look different than I remember!* Maybe you noticed a new wrinkle, more gray hair, a furrowed brow from aches in your body. You can't deny it—you are getting older. But you are not alone. Many adults experience age-based discrimination, and this impacts physical and mental health,[35] adding to the pressure you already feel. Don't let growing older get you down; life is in a constant state of change. Defy expectations and inspire others by being authentic to your true self. Focus on living with joy and happiness no matter how old you are.

*I always have the power to inspire others
and embark on creative new adventures.
It is never too late to explore the things
I am passionate about.*

RESTFUL RITUAL

Get excited for the next chapter of your life—start dreaming *before* your head hits the pillow! What new learning experience, hobby, or meet-up group can you join? Commit to signing up this week.

I SEE THINGS FOR WHAT THEY ARE, NOT WHAT I THINK THEY SHOULD BE.

Are you pretending things are better than they actually are? Sometimes we focus on potential or live in a fantasy instead of taking situations at face value. Tonight, take a life inventory, looking at all the areas where you are wearing rose-colored glasses or putting on a brave face. Be honest with yourself so that you can be more honest with those around you. Give yourself permission to look at things as they are instead of how you wish they were. Acceptance is the key to freedom from disappointment and past outcomes.

I do not force, change, or try to fix what I cannot. I take full responsibility for looking at my life the way it is right now and let go of the past. From this place of full acceptance, I align with desirable outcomes.

RESTFUL RITUAL

Take a rose petal aromatherapy bath before bed. Remove the petals from one or two organic (free of pesticides) roses, or use rose essential oil. Add the petals to your bath water, and soak in bliss.

I HEAL WHAT I AM WILLING TO REVEAL.

Where does most of your stress come from? The people in your life can add stress by complaining, gossiping, and demanding things from you, but sometimes the most stressful person in your life is you. We don't always recognize our own unhealthy habits or toxic traits—what if *we* are the negative drama llama?! It's easy to blame others for your unhappiness, but if you keep finding yourself in the same types of situations with different people, the common connector might be you. You are either allowing the behavior from others, or you are creating them. Your behaviors, perspective, and choices are either creating more stress in your life or bringing more peace. Tonight, be self-aware: look at the stuck patterns hindering your growth. Be willing to shake up and release them, so you can heal.

What stays is meant for me, and what leaves is meant to be free. I let things go, because I am in flow.

RESTFUL RITUAL

Free your body to induce quality sleep. Stand up and shake your entire body, rocking, jumping, moving back and forth and side to side. This shaking releases trauma and stuck energy.

I CONCLUDE MY DAY WITH LOVE IN MY HEART.

We all have insecurities and fears that hold us back, making life harder than it needs to be. The reality is that you are loved no matter what, regardless of these fears. Staying trapped in self-doubt keeps you playing small in life. If you have a hard time releasing your doubt, recognize that self-doubt is just your ego mind projecting its deepest fears to protect itself from the unknown. Strengthen your self-worth by taking time each night to reflect on the things you are grateful for about your life and yourself, big or small.

I am stronger than my doubts. I believe in myself and my abilities, and I am proud of who I am. I am loved beyond measure and share the gift of love with myself.

RESTFUL RITUAL

Focus on love as you prepare for bed. Place a rose quartz crystal in a sacred space in your bedroom to evoke compassion and heart healing in the entire room.

I GO WITH THE FLOW.

Make a practice of going with the flow in all areas of your life. This does not mean that you allow mistreatment or disrespect at your own expense; rather, this concept focuses on energy. Look at the energy of the people, situations, opportunities, and experiences around you and ask, *Does this feel in alignment with me?* When we work with the flow of life, we tap into a greater support from the universe. There is a natural vibrational frequency that matches yours—this is how the law of attraction works. Your thoughts create results. Focus on what you want and allow it to come to you, with effortless flow and joyful ease.

I go with the flow by trusting the universe—
I do not force outcomes. Relaxation and peace
reside in the natural unfolding of my life.

RESTFUL RITUAL

Do some reflection before bed. Pour yourself a glass of filtered water or herbal tea and sip it while you journal on an outcome of your life that you're trying to force instead of flowing with it.

I CONNECT WITH MY INNER CHILD THROUGH COMPASSION AND JOY.

What did you spend most of your playtime doing as a child? In the adult world, it's even more important to maintain that childlike sense of wonder—nothing challenges joy more than the weight of grown-up expectations. It's also normal if you had an imaginary friend who provided companionship, especially in times of loneliness, distress, and transition—a need that continues into adulthood. Reflect on your childhood and the coping mechanisms that calmed you; you are your inner child's companion now. In times of stress, return to the simplicity of your younger years.

I explore the imagination of my inner child.
I think less so I can play more. Our safe space
is a joyful place.

RESTFUL RITUAL

Invite a carefree vibe to your sleep tonight with the happy baby yoga pose: Lay on your back and bring your knees to either side of your chest, holding the bottoms of your feet and gently rocking from side to side. Stay in this position for several deep and joyful breaths.

I ASCEND WITH WISDOM AND COMPASSION.

Many of us have baseline emotions—feelings we resort to—to avoid less desirable feelings. How do you handle stressful situations? You always have a choice: proactivity or reactivity. If you are prone to the latter, choose to respond in a new way—with poise and compassion. Ask yourself, *Is this response true to my feelings?* Perhaps your anger masks shame. Shift your energy to a higher vibration, and welcome the lesson that needs to be learned; shed the patterns of the past and ascend. Emotions are fleeting and unreliable when left unchecked. Practice self-compassion as you free yourself from what no longer serves you. Return to inner balance and wisdom.

I am balanced in my head and heart, and I welcome what shows up there. I respond with wisdom and compassion.

RESTFUL RITUAL

Do an emotional cleanse to usher in peaceful sleep. Put on your earphones and play one of your moodiest, saddest songs. Let yourself feel all the feels, and cry if you need to cry—let it all out with abandon.

I HONOR MY NEED TO BELONG BY ALIGNING WITH KINDRED SPIRITS.

If you frequently find yourself in situations where you don't feel like you fit in, were aspects of your childhood the same? Did you grow up feeling invalidated—perhaps at home or in school by people who made you feel like an outsider? This may have given you an independent nature, but there's more going on: a deep, inner longing for belonging. This desire could be the undertone of most of your interactions now. If you've been feeling lonely, give yourself the gift of an inner circle of like minds and hearts. Seek a supportive network of kindred spirits who honor that inner need. You deserve to be surrounded by people who love you for being *you*.

I am my own best friend, and I know there are people out there for me. I cherish my relationships and tend to them with care.

RESTFUL RITUAL

Tonight, think about someone you'd like to get to know better, and make a friend date to get together with them this week.

I EXAMINE MY FRUSTRATIONS AND TRUST THE DIVINE FLOW.

So often, we run from the uncomfortable aspects of life, but there is a reason that certain things bother you—pay attention! When you try to escape triggering situations rather than addressing them, it perpetuates a stunted growth cycle. Spiritual bypassing is the tendency to skip over or avoid facing unresolved emotional issues—does this resonate with your behavior? Healing is needed for you to move into the next phase of your life. Let your frustrations teach you and guide you forward. From this place of clarity, you'll find solutions that align with you.

I receive inspired guidance daily and trust the divine flow of my life. I view problems as opportunities to find solutions.

RESTFUL RITUAL

Before bed, stretch your body. Focus on a tight muscle and gently force it into a sustained stretch. Within your own window of tolerance, stay present with the uncomfortable sensations that come up, then offer gratitude for the feelings of comfort when you release. Do the same with difficult thoughts and emotions if they arise this week.

I AM HERE, IN THIS MOMENT, EMBRACING WHAT IS.

We live in such a busy, chaotic world that being able to turn off the go-go-go energy is essential. Practicing mindfulness and presence in the moment is one of the best tools you can use to give your body and mind some reprieve. If you struggle with relaxing and find it hard to slow down, focus on the moment by using all your physical senses. Return to the grounding space of your body as you pay attention to your surroundings: What do you see? What do you hear? What can you touch? What can you smell? Your experience in the present space offers peace. Take this time to embrace it.

All I really have is right here in this moment; in it, I am safe, secure, and free of frustrations and distractions.

RESTFUL RITUAL

As you prepare for sleep, focus fully on this moment by engaging all of your senses—what do you see, feel (touch), hear, taste, smell? Which of these senses resonates most with you? Return to it for additional grounding.

I TAKE COURAGEOUS CHANCES ON MYSELF.

There are people who have ten-year plans mapped out and vision boards laminated and pinned up, and then there are those who don't even know what they'll eat for dinner tonight. If you relate to the latter, you could be so tuned in to what's happening now that you don't spend enough time thinking about the future. Staying in the present moment is admirable, but be honest with yourself: Are you living intentionally or haphazardly, with no clear direction? While nobody can predict the future, you *can* shape it by getting in touch with your heart's deepest desires. Take a chance on you! Be bold and brave! Say yes to using your time wisely and making the most of your time on Earth.

I have so much to offer this world—I have a unique purpose. I foster this by infusing my heart's desires with wisdom and intention. I show up courageously for me.

RESTFUL RITUAL

Tonight, jumpstart your goals by starting or adding to your vision board, either digitally (with Canva or Pinterest) or physically (with magazines).

I CELEBRATE ALL THE POSITIVE POSSIBILITIES.

There's a whole new life experience waiting for you—untapped, unseen, and unbeknownst to you—and it's just around the corner! It's possible that your current situation (home, job, partner) has become too comfortable and growth is no longer an option; it may be time to release yourself to move in a new direction. The same is true when things become so uncomfortable that staying takes too much out of us—leaving becomes the only choice. Give yourself permission to expand into the possibilities waiting for you. Say yes, take that next step forward, and embrace the new chapters unfolding in your life.

I release any area in my life that feels restricted, forced, uncomfortable, unmanageable, or complacent. I let myself grow into the new phases of my life with honesty, courage, and a dedication to aligning to my true self.

RESTFUL RITUAL

Tonight, step into dreamland *before* you fall asleep. Visualize yourself living the life you truly want and experiencing your ideal day. What does it look like? How does it feel?

QUALITY SLEEP RESTORES MY STRENGTH.

Sleep architecture is the structure of sleep you get each night. There are two types of sleep—nonrapid eye movement (NREM) and rapid eye movement (REM) sleep—and four distinct stages, with stages three and four being the deepest. Stage four of deep sleep (REM) is essential for your body and brain, as this stage supports tissue repair and hormone regulation and gives your brain an opportunity to clear waste. If you toss and turn at night, get up a lot to go to the bathroom, and wake up feeling tired, you most likely did not get enough of these final two stages. Not getting enough deep sleep may cause migraines[36] and can decrease mental sharpness, along with other cognitive issues with memory and learning.[37] Start prioritizing quality sleep tonight.

I bask in the energy of deep rest. My strength is restored and my spirit renewed.

RESTFUL RITUAL

Prepare tonight to start tracking your sleep. Leave a journal by your bed to record duration and quality in the morning. (You could also invest in a sleep-tracking device.)

I LEAN INTO MY FAITH– IT FREES ME FROM FEAR.

Anxiety gets a bad reputation, but it's a valuable indicator of what needs more attention and balance in your life. Anxiety happens when worst-case scenarios pop into your head and create catastrophic thoughts. It's your body's way of saying, *Stranger danger!* But sometimes that stranger who's causing the most stress is *you*. Do you panic because you don't trust yourself or fear the unknown future? Do you think you have the capacity or capability to handle the outcome? Remember you are always enough and fully able—attune with this belief above all. You'll never be given more than you can handle.

I free myself from anxiety with faith in myself and my capabilities. I am strong and resilient, and I handle all situations with grace and ease.

RESTFUL RITUAL

Massage your temples to invite rest tonight. Close your eyes, and move your fingers in a clockwise motion for five to ten seconds; reverse the motion for another five to ten seconds. Do this a few times, until you drop into your body and feel calm.

MY ENERGY PROTECTS ME FROM STRESS.

Your body is an energy magnet surrounded by a force field of protection—your aura. When you are depleted and tired, however, it can be easier for negative things (thoughts, other people's agendas, fears, and disease) to leak in and get you down. In contrast, when you're balanced and well rested, you're stronger, healthier, happier, and less bothered. Take an inventory of your day: Did you give beyond your capacity or have major lapses in energy? Are you ruminating over something frustrating that happened? If so, your aura may have holes in it. Patch yourself up with self-protection and self-care. It is important to protect your energetic field and clear it regularly.

I honor my aura and its protective energy by releasing stress and negativity. I allow myself to rest and recharge to restore its power.

RESTFUL RITUAL

Cleanse your aura before bed with a selenite crystal (wand). Hold the crystal about five inches away from your body and sweep it from head to toe, visualizing all negative energy being removed from your body.

I FIND POWER AND CLARITY IN MY STILLNESS.

Many of us are conditioned to be superhuman—to be pleasant on the surface and do good deeds no matter what. We push ourselves to the limit and do it all without complaining, but it's not normal or healthy to ignore your limits—no one person can take on the entire world. The pressure you've been carrying around is too heavy and eventually leads to collapse. It's time to release the pressure, slow down, and find safety and clarity in stillness.

I dare to live my life in a relaxed way.
I actively participate in rest by choosing
to quiet my mind and listen to the still,
small voice within.

RESTFUL RITUAL

Tonight, practice circular breathing: Close your eyes and breathe into your body through your nose. As you exhale through your mouth, let the circular cadence of your breathing go in and out for three to five seconds on each inhale and exhale. As you breathe, stand and sway or hug yourself. It's a great way to self-soothe and self-regulate.

I SUPPORT MYSELF TO BETTER SUPPORT OTHERS.

If things are uncertain in your life, it can be hard to relax. It's extra difficult to calm the mind when situations around you feel unmanageable or inescapable. Perhaps you're dealing with supporting another (a child, an aging parent, a senior pet); there are phases in our lives when the needs of others are our responsibility. The stability of those you love and care for is a priority, yet finding balance in these situations is essential to your own well-being. If you're having a difficult time with this, focus on doing one small thing for yourself every day. Supporting others requires us to support ourselves when we can, one moment at a time.

I modify my self-care routine so I can still show up for myself, especially when others need me. The better I care for myself, the better I can care for them.

RESTFUL RITUAL

Wind down tonight by making a lavender sachet. Put dried lavender with a couple drops of lavender oil into a cotton or linen sachet, and place it under your pillow.

I PRACTICE SELF-LOVE BY GIVING MYSELF REST.

You are doing amazing at life. When is the last time you really looked in the mirror and said, "I've got this! I am awesome! I'm so proud of me!" So often, we don't stop to think about the good that we're doing; we're usually so busy focusing on others and taking care of them that it actually seems selfish to turn our attention inward. What are *your* needs? What is precious to *you*? Relax and rest into this moment with more peace and serenity as you give yourself a generous helping of the love and gratitude you so willingly give away.

I am proud of me and how far I've come.
I claim the personal time I deserve,
starting with quality rest.

RESTFUL RITUAL

Get your glow on with a face mask tonight. If you don't have one, create your own deep-cleansing mud mask: mix two tablespoons of powdered clay, one tablespoon of aloe vera gel, and two to three drops of lavender (or your favorite) essential oil. Rub it on your face, let it dry for 10–15 minutes, and rinse off with warm water. As you rinse off the mask repeat tonight's mantra.

I TREAT MY ENTIRE BEING WITH RESPECT.

Where are you spending most of your time and energy? Maybe you prioritize your health by taking care of your body with movement and quality foods, but you criticize and judge yourself harshly. When you do this, you create an imbalance within you. If you truly value your health, make sure you include your *whole* self. The foods you eat and your self-talk impact your sleep for better or worse too. Choose foods and words that are nutritious and supportive, making you feel good inside and out. Treat your entire being with respect, because you are worth it.

I value all layers of my life—my mental,
spiritual, physical, and emotional well-being.
I am well when I am in balance.

RESTFUL RITUAL

Take time before bed to make a sleep-friendly meal plan for the week. Embrace whole grains, lean proteins, heart-healthy fats, fresh herbs, and foods high in magnesium, and eat two to four hours before bedtime. Drinking an adaptogen tea prior to bed (made with herbs like ashwagandha or ginseng)[38] is also helpful.

I AM LOYAL TO MY UNIQUE NATURE.

It is exhausting to be stuck in your head, battling what you *should* do versus what you *want* to do. Do you give away your power to an outside authority? Do you bend to the demands and wishes of others easily? Our inner autonomy is diminished when we outsource our direction and give others the keys to our happiness. Trust yourself and your innate ability to make choices that fit with your true self. Take tonight as an opportunity to reflect on how aligned you feel your life is. Let go of the demands of others and relax into following your own true path.

*I do not let the pressure of others'
demands and wishes affect my autonomy.
I acknowledge my innate inner authority and
true self. I am my own champion, creating the
life that is right for me.*

RESTFUL RITUAL

Before bed tonight, start a special box for your secret dreams, goals, and desires, making a ceremony of writing them down on paper and placing them into your sacred box for safekeeping.

I PROTECT MY ENERGY AND ALIGN TO WHAT RESONATES WITH ME.

It's your role to protect your energy and kindness from those who do not see your value. When you give and receive openly to those who return the same, you have more energy; but when you give to people who only take, it depletes your energy. Protect your energy by being your own fierce protector. Keep it shielded from people who do not have the best intentions for you. Be consciously aware that your uplifting energy attracts all kinds of people. What types of people are you allowing into your life? Choose reciprocal relationships that fill your love cup and add to your energy, not deplete it.

My energy is essential to my life—it is sacred. I protect this energy by aligning to people and circumstances that best support and enrich it.

RESTFUL RITUAL

Lighten your sleep atmosphere by using rhythm and frequency to cleanse your bedroom space tonight. Use crystal bowls, bells, tuning forks, or a sound-healing meditation from online—pick whatever resonates with you.

I HONOR MY SADNESS TONIGHT.

It's easy to get stuck in a deep well of heavy emotions when we don't allow ourselves to feel or express them. Do you have emotions that you are avoiding? Sadness, grief, shame—there are many unpleasant emotions that we are afraid to feel, perhaps because we have stuffed them down so deeply we fear a tsunami of uncontrolled energy if we go there. Tonight is a reminder that you are safe to feel what you need to feel. Instead of freezing up and turning away from healing, dive into the sadness to rise back to the surface—back to your true and perfect self.

I embrace my feelings, allowing them to be as they are. My emotional needs matter, and I express them fully. I honor my feelings and trust myself to care for them.

RESTFUL RITUAL

Send yourself to sleep with a butterfly hug—a somatic exercise for self-soothing. Wrap your arms around your body and hold yourself like you would hold a dear friend you love and accept unconditionally.

I GIVE UP THE GOOD AND GO FOR THE GREAT.

Are you settling? Sometimes we convince ourselves things are better than they actually are. Are you just taking what life has given you, allowing it to be what it is, or are you focusing on pursuing what you truly want? So often, we settle because we think we don't deserve better. Or we stick with what seems good when we can really aim for great. Use tonight as a reminder that you have more to live for and in your heart than has been actualized. If you want to live a meaningful life, going for great requires courage, honesty, and a steadfast commitment to honoring your true self and your heart. Trust that you already have what it takes within you.

I am all I need, and I give myself permission to embrace all of me. I go for what I want beyond what I have lived.

RESTFUL RITUAL

Activate your imagination before falling asleep. Take your index finger on your dominant hand and tap the third-eye space above your nose, in between both of your eyes. Do this ten to fifteen times, playing with the energy of what could be.

I DESERVE A LIFE OF HAPPINESS, MEANING, AND JOY.

Look around you at all the things going well in your beautiful life—you can always access more meaning and joy by paying attention to what happiness means to you. Sometimes we feel like we don't deserve the good things that are meant for us because others are suffering, or because we are unworthy. If you feel this way, focus for a minute on gratitude, taking in the abundance that is available to you. In this energy, you start to open yourself up to new possibilities and realize that you deserve all the amazing things that are on their way to you.

I feel alive and vibrant—I deserve to be happy. The more energy I give to the appreciation of my life, the more happiness and joy I experience.

RESTFUL RITUAL

As you get settled in bed tonight, investigate your sleep environment, considering ways to upgrade it. Invest in new pillows, sheets, or blankets or some other comfort to make bedtime more inviting.

I OPEN MYSELF TO RECEIVE WHAT I CANNOT YET CONCEIVE.

Being able to receive is one of the most important life skills you can have. Not only does it help you feel more balanced, but it satisfies the innate need to feel validated, seen, and recognized. Are you open to receiving what you've been able to give? Being able to receive also means expanding our conception of the amount of abundance and support available to us, especially when we've been so focused on giving to others. It's time to pull back your energy and let others help you—you don't have to do it all alone. Asking for help is not a weakness; it is your greatest strength.

I open myself to others' support to reduce stress and find balance. I allow myself to receive all the things I have yet to conceive, for the universe knows what serves my highest good.

RESTFUL RITUAL

Clear your mental space before bed by identifying a situation causing you stress. Ask your guides, the universe, the divine for what you need, and then release the stress to their care.

My steadfast gratitude attracts abundance.

Each day brings new opportunities for us to practice gratitude, and sometimes it's through trials and tribulations. If your life has been turned upside down by a surprising or traumatic event, it can be impossible for you to focus on anything but the situation immediately at hand. Whether it's a diagnosis of a disease, financial troubles, or an unexpected divorce, this devastation can implode your world. Situations like this are impossible to handle if you're not appreciating what is still going *well*. No matter what you're going through, recognize the simple joys all around you. Navigate life's troubles with more grace and ease by turning to gratitude and your life's unshakable abundance.

Whatever life throws at me, I am comfortable to catch it. I am grateful through it all— gratitude and abundance are my anchors.

Restful Ritual

Before bed, enter into a space of gratitude and peace. Make a list in your journal of what you are most grateful for from today. You can place the list under your pillow before you fall asleep to invite in more peaceful dreams.

I RELEASE LIMITING BELIEFS AND STORIES.

Does this sound familiar? The popular girl from high school just posted another photo on social media of her way-too-gorgeous family, and you think to yourself, *I can't even get my kids dressed without a raging tantrum!* Who has time for perfected poses when you're scrambling daily to make sure laundry's done, veggies are eaten, pets are walked? "Mom guilt" is a real thing, and you don't have to be female or a mother to experience it. Comparing yourself to others in any manner is an insidious cycle of self-blame that leads nowhere. Tonight, give yourself more credit—you're doing a great job! Take some time to celebrate and care for *you*.

*I release myself from past mistakes,
all perceived flaws, and unrealistic
expectations—I release limiting thoughts
that I am not good enough or doing enough.
Every day, I do my best, and it is enough.*

RESTFUL RITUAL

Letting go is your only agenda tonight! Practice being in the moment through your sense of taste. Take a chunk from your favorite bar of dark chocolate and enjoy it free of guilt. Let go of any worry, as you mindfully embrace the moment.

I EMBRACE THE MOON'S MEDICINE—NEW CYCLES OF AWARENESS AND GROWTH.

The nighttime brings a slowing down; its blanket of darkness and peace offering a new opportunity for us to go inward and reflect on the conscious creation of our deepest desires. When you dream at night, you're able to manifest a deeper level of self-awareness. The moon is a powerful manifestation tool, with its allure of divine feminine power and illumination; it gives us an opportunity to find truth and clarity. Each phase of the moon is unique—a multitude of numerous energies and benefits; when was the last time you looked up to travel within? As the moon watches over you tonight, connect with its power to dive deeper into your heart's wisdom and desires.

In the stillness and peace of night, I cultivate a deeper sense of self-awareness with the moon as my guiding light.

RESTFUL RITUAL

Before bed, ask the moon for guidance: "Moon, what medicine do you have for me tonight?" Open your awareness, and listen with your heart for the answer.

221

I AM PROUD OF MYSELF FOR TRYING.

When you go for your dreams and follow your heart, all should turn out the way you hope, right? This is the perspective we hold dear; however, there's a bigger picture at play. The choices you make from your heart are never wrong, and going for what you want is what a deeper life experience is all about; yet the outcome is not as important as the journey. Don't look back and regret your choices. If you're in a situation right now that didn't go as expected, just recognize that your expectations are what limit you, not your dreams. Be proud of yourself for trying, because what you went through is exactly what you needed to learn the lessons for next time.

I make choices with my heart and welcome the wisdom of my life experiences. I align with directions that resonate with my highest self.

RESTFUL RITUAL

In your journal tonight, trace the lineage of a disappointment from its place in the past to the present: How has your life evolved since? What skills have been strengthened?

I SAIL THROUGH LIFE'S CHANGES WITH GRACE AND EASE.

Change is inevitable—something that happens to all of us every day and at multiple stages in our lives (adolescence, adulthood, parenthood, retirement, etc.). No matter what, navigating change is easier with grace. Within all the choices you make, forge the path forward with inspiration and joy in your heart. When you do this, you will feel more alive and free; you will no longer rest in your anxieties and fears, because you will be so connected to your truth that change will no longer stunt you. Make the changes you are going through easier by infusing change with grace, love, and appreciation.

I am the master changemaker of my life. I embrace change with love and grace—this is my source of power.

RESTFUL RITUAL

Cold water therapy is great at helping to release anxiety and stress. Tonight, consider taking a cool shower or giving yourself an ice-water facial. Fill a large bowl with water and ice and submerge your face for 10–15 seconds at a time for 3–5 minutes. This can jump-start your system back into peace and presence for a good night's sleep.

DISAPPOINTMENTS ARE MY GREATEST TEACHERS.

Does it seem like others constantly let you down and you can't trust anyone? Do you secretly fear you will never be happy? We all have deep-seated secrets that we hide from others and even ourselves. We assume keeping quiet keeps us safe, but most of the time, secrets hold us back. Grow beyond the limitations of your unconscious fears by looking at your life and mental health like an onion, always peeling back new layers—there's always more to learn and heal. Tonight, take an inventory of what has disappointed you the most in your life. Infuse more love into all of your disappointments, and accept the lessons they offer.

I appreciate all the experiences that I've had—they are my greatest teachers. The lessons I have learned create a more successful present and future.

RESTFUL RITUAL

Before bed, take out your journal and jot down things or people you've been disappointed by, symbolically removing them from your mind. Next to each disappointment, write a lesson learned from each experience, and release it with love.

I AM A GOOD PERSON.

We've all had moments where we harmed others out of self-protection. Much like a child who has not yet learned accountability and self-awareness in their interactions, we may try to push boundaries and lie, to see what we can get away with (thoughts like, *If I don't look at the truth, then maybe it doesn't exist*). But the truth is always the way to go. Be honest about where you are lying to yourself or hiding behind half-truths. When your inner child lives the *I am not enough lie*, step into the light of your confident self: *I am an awesome person*. Trust the truth: you are good. Let your stunning self lead the way.

I live my truth—I am a good person—and I honor the good in others when I do.

RESTFUL RITUAL

In your journal tonight, reflect on a failure that still haunts you. What is the story you tell yourself about this mistake? Now ask yourself about the "secret success" that came out of the experience.

I RISE TO THIS OCCASION, FOR I HAVE STRENGTH BEYOND MEASURE.

Are you simply doing the best you can to make it through, yet life keeps throwing you obstacle after obstacle? The reality is, you're not a victim to the circumstances of your own life; you're in warrior training—you're stronger than you give yourself credit for. These things happen so we can dig deeper into this inner strength; in hard times, we find out what we are made of and discover depths to our character. Be kind to yourself, be gentle with yourself, believe in yourself. When you activate the warrior within, you rise up with greater strength and inner power, ready for whatever comes your way.

I rise above each challenge, higher and higher, for I am a warrior—a defender of my unique strengths. I am victorious in my life's opportunities.

RESTFUL RITUAL

Victory power pose! Before bed tonight, stand up with your hands in a V shape above your head. Radiate there in all your glory, drawing energy through your limbs and into your chest and heart.

REST IS ESSENTIAL TO MY BODY, MIND, AND SOUL.

Your body is always talking to you—are you listening? Often, when we think we should "just power through," what our body really needs is rest. Taking time to rest brings you back into optimal balance. Start preparing for a better night's sleep by listening to your body during the day. If you feel a nap is needed, honor your body. Studies show daytime napping can improve cognitive function.[39] Especially for shift workers, naps have the power to improve reaction time and alertness. While quality sleep at night is the ultimate goal, the occasional boost of a nap can go a long way.

When I prioritize rest, I take my life into my own hands. I am in control of how I show up in all situations, physically, mentally, and spiritually.

RESTFUL RITUAL

Tonight, make a mindful plan for times when you need a healthy boost. For example, you could take a siesta power nap (ten to fifteen minutes) in the afternoon. Getting up and stretching is always helpful too.

Disruptive thoughts do not disturb my peace.

What is the difference between stress and anxiety? Stress is caused by something external, whereas anxiety is internal—your inner dialog and feelings. Both are responses to your brain's belief that you are in danger; and both cause apprehension, body aches, and loss of sleep. If you feel overwhelmed by emotions and feel a sense of danger you may fall into a fight-or-flight response, which is also called the "amygdala hijack." When we feel unsafe, our amygdala (the part of your brain that processes emotions and responses) goes into defense mode, then responds with a fight for survival or attempt to flee to find safety.[40] Not everything is a threat, however; the influence of past traumatic experiences evokes an exaggerated stress response. Learn to discern the difference by bringing yourself back to the present—it will never lead you astray.

I live in the present to maneuver the pains of the past. I am calm, safe, and balanced.

Restful Ritual

Focus on grounding before bed. Choose an object in your home that you can dedicate as a source of safety and calm. This week, every time you walk by it, touch it while saying out loud "calm" and "safe." Make this item a reference point in your mind's eye too, calling on it whenever necessary.

THE GIFTS OF LIFE
ARE WITHIN ME.

Your life is so precious—a true gift. It can be hard to recognize how important your life is when you're overwhelmed by daily demands and expectations. What's easy is getting caught up in the frustrations of life, such as paying bills, doing chores, fixing things—all of which can become exhausting. Remember that within you are innate skills that can help you navigate each situation with more ease—breath, peace, creativity, calm—not to mention your one-of-a-kind talents that make you *you*. Relax into the simple pleasures of life knowing that *you've got this*. Allow yourself to express the gifts and talents that are already within you.

I am comfortable in my body in this moment, here and now. I utilize and honor my innate gifts by living each day from the inside out.

RESTFUL RITUAL

Tonight, moisturize your entire body with your favorite lotion as you appreciate your natural gifts and talents. Tuck yourself into bed feeling cared for, honored, and loved.

REST AND LOVE ARE MY PERFECT DESTINATIONS.

All is well when we relax into our divine state—the loving presence within. When you detach from the outside world and return to your inner world, you realize that you are always resting in love; and love is the answer to all. Think of it as a staycation—there's no need to force or push yourself into achieving anything; love is enough. If you're feeling stuck in any area of your life, fear may be at fault. Take a look at your actions and motivations, and redirect your attention to love. Let the compassion and purpose within guide you forward.

I allow the love within to flow through me and out into the world. When I access this love, I access the perfection of the moment. Everything, as it is, is meant to be.

RESTFUL RITUAL

Tonight, make time for love. Schedule sexy time with your partner (or yourself, if flying solo). The release of oxytocin, the "love hormone," can promote relaxation and a sense of well-being. Plus, kissing and cuddling fosters emotional connection.

My life is beautiful, every day.

Your life is a series of mini events creating extraordinary results. So often, we feel like we need to achieve more than what we already have. We may have a big benchmark or specific thing in our mind that we are working toward—the pressure and expectations we put on ourselves are enormous. Each day may be about manifesting new goals, but your life is not just one big manifestation after another; it's actually the smaller moments in between that make up the most miraculous memories. Your life is beautiful today, in this moment, and the next, and the next after that. Give yourself permission and space to celebrate this extraordinary gift.

My life is a beautiful manifestation of all my thoughts, desires, and goals. I celebrate it and my ever-expanding growth.

Restful Ritual

In preparation for rest, snuggle down in bed with a pile of pillows, blankets, and gratitude. Lie in wonderment and awe of the beautiful aspects of your life, and fall to sleep with a smile.

I TRUST MYSELF AND MY RHYTHM.

Do you stop before you start or before you finish? Do you tend to self-sabotage good opportunities? The foundation for any healthy relationship is trust, even with oneself. Without faith in yourself, it's impossible to move forward on any goal or dream. Whether you ignore your intuition, outsource advice, procrastinate, or ruminate on past choices, it all comes back to not recognizing your own value—to not trusting yourself! Detach from the programming and codependency of the outside world to stand in your truth—this is how your soul grows. Trust yourself—according to the rhythm within.

I live by the pace of my own rhythm and dreams. I trust myself and my worth, regulating my inner world to maintain balance, no matter what my outer circumstances.

RESTFUL RITUAL

Set aside some quiet time before bed. With your eyes closed, observe where in your life societal expectations and external pressures have kept you from being your authentic self. Make a commitment to trust and honor yourself more, from this moment on.

I SET MY FOCUS AND IMAGINATION ON PROFOUND LOVE.

There's a higher love available to you when you do the necessary inner work. Your life is filled with opportunities for self-reflection and personal development, and love is your greatest teacher. Give yourself permission to receive love from the universe and from others. If you've closed off or resented certain people because of things they were unable to give, forgive them and allow yourself to feel whatever you needed from them. Open up to more love, hand your troubles over to the universe, and trust that all is in right order. When you align with love, everything flourishes.

I am loving, I am loved, I am lovable. I give and receive from the unlimited love of Source. All is available to me, and a higher love is what I desire.

RESTFUL RITUAL

Make a love to-do list before bed—who have you lost touch with and who have you been missing? This week, commit to telling at least one person that you love them without expecting to hear anything in return.

I HONOR MY LIFE'S JOURNEY AS A BEAUTIFUL WORK IN PROGRESS.

Ahh, it feels good to do the work and heal. Reading self-help books, watching TEDx talks, listening to podcasts, working with your coaches—look at you go! Just remember to check in with yourself along the way: Are you appreciating the shifts in your life? Do you see how you handle problems differently than you used to? How your emotions are more regulated? How you've forgiven yourself? The healing journey is not linear, nor is it ever complete. You may be intellectualizing your healing but not fully embodying all the concepts you're learning. Take some time to integrate what you have learned so far and honor yourself in the process.

All I've been through is part of my greater
purpose and plan—I am healing and growing.
I integrate and embody these lessons in
my ever-evolving self.

RESTFUL RITUAL

The close of this day calls for some celebration—you're living your best life! Savor a favorite treat in your honor, taking in peace and satisfaction with each bite.

I TRUST IN THE STRENGTH AND SECURITY OF MY EMOTIONAL BONDS.

Are you romanticizing a relationship, focusing on how things *could be* versus paying attention to how they really are? Once a person is close enough for real intimacy, do you pull back and detach? This could be an avoidant attachment style, the opposite of an anxious or preoccupied attachment style, and it causes a sense of betrayal in any relationship dynamic. Fear is usually preventing us from leaning into love, but at our core, we are all hardwired for connection. Whether you relate with the avoidant pattern or the anxious attachment style, focus on healing the original attachment wound, so you may find security in yourself and all of your relationships.

I am brave, reaching out to others when I want to withdraw. Even when I'm afraid, I lean on the power of love to build strong emotional bonds.

RESTFUL RITUAL

Practice vulnerability as your bedtime exercise. Reach out to a friend or spend some quality time with your partner (or loved one) with the intention of sharing something that's been weighing on your heart.

When I rest, I reset.

If you've had a day that really worked you over, resetting yourself is the most important thing you can do. Start the minute you get settled at home, nourishing your body with a healthy meal. Return to the calm of the present moment with mindful eating, opening your senses to the experience and activating a deep sense of rest. Turn off the news and television, and tune out all other distractions as you prepare for bed. Create a restorative atmosphere outside to support the night's restoration inside.

As I rest, I reset mentally, physically, and spiritually. I prioritize rest with the time and self-love I require to restore myself fully.

Restful Ritual

Concentrate on releasing pressure and anxiety by squeezing a stress ball or working a piece of clay or Silly Putty before bed. Identify a situation that's troubling you, and use your breath to infuse it with calm. Imagine expelling this energy with every exhale, as you squeeze, until the problem feels released and at peace.

THERE IS NOWHERE ELSE I WOULD RATHER BE.

It may feel like you are going off track, but consider this: What if you're simply making an adjustment on the road of your highest good? There are forces at work that are bigger and brighter than you can imagine—surrender yourself to them. Embrace the life that is working to emerge. The redirected path *is* your path—it will always lead you in the right direction. Your higher power would never put you in a position that is not in your best interest. Recognize that where you are is exactly where you're supposed to be. With your soul in the driver's seat, all is in divine order.

I live in accordance with my own heart, and the world adjusts accordingly. I am right where I'm supposed to be.

RESTFUL RITUAL

Tonight, try this stress-relieving exercise: lie on your back, move your bum as close to the wall as possible, and put your legs up, so they're supported against the wall. Legs up the wall pose is good for relaxation and stress relief. Stay in this position for as long as it feels good.

I take full responsibility for all my experiences.

Does it seem like bad things keep happening to you? At this point, you might be thinking, *I can't do anything about it, so why even try?* If this is your mindset, you are trapped in negative self-talk, self-sabotage, and a victim mentality—a feeling that you have no personal power and are at the whim of external situations. Ask yourself, *Do I feel safer in this energy of lack because I fear disappointment? Do I believe I deserve happiness?* Your intrinsic value does not come from external experiences, mistakes, or the ways others treat you—you're designed to be happy. Take accountability for it. Get out of your own way to claim this birthright.

Everything I experience—pleasant or not—is part of my joyful journey. I embrace every opportunity to expand and grow.

Restful Ritual

Before bed, light a candle, and in your journal, write down what a victim mindset is costing you. When you're ready to blow out the candle, imagine blowing the resentment away forever, leaving only peace in your heart.

I ADD IMMENSE VALUE TO THE WORLD.

You are enough, and you have great value to share with others. Your worth does not come from your achievements, social media posts, what you do, how much money you have in the bank, or who you are married to. If you are chasing approval, it could be because you don't feel confident at your core. You hide your true self from others as well as yourself, and this causes discomfort within. Take some time this evening to really align with your personal preferences. What is important to *you*? When you start to live according to these standards, you become more valuable to yourself and the world.

I show my true self to others and celebrate my differences. What makes me unique is what makes me valuable.

RESTFUL RITUAL

Before bed, concentrate on moisturizing your feet with intention. As you massage your toes, heels, soles, and the tops of your feet, thank them for taking you where you need to go in the world.

I AM A PEACEFUL SLEEPER.

Sleeping peacefully at night is a beautiful gift to yourself, your body, and your spirit. When you go to bed and relax your entire being, your soul has the opportunity to escape the everyday world—to drift off into dreamland. As you visit other realms and explore new possibilities there, you expand your entire aura—the unseen field of energy around you. And when you wake up, you feel more refreshed and connected to your surroundings and all their inhabitants. Imagine that when you're asleep, you're connected to a collective energy of oneness, peace, and happiness that is available to all. Peace on Earth is possible; start tonight in your dreams.

I choose to embody and sleep in a peaceful, restorative state. Peace is my priority every night, and I set myself up for quality sleep.

RESTFUL RITUAL

Support a peaceful sleep tonight by cueing up a deep-sleep meditation on Spotify, YouTube, SoundCloud, or another meditation resource and drift asleep under its guidance.

Tranquility balances my life and my mood.

Reflect on your emotional experiences throughout the day. Did you feel connected to yourself and productive—in the zone? Did you experience any sudden disruptions that shifted you into a state of anger, frustration, or despair? Riding waves of emotions is part of living a balanced life; getting swept away by them creates imbalance. Acknowledging each emotion is important when trying to maintain a centered state, especially as you transition from your day into your night. Do you have unresolved issues or unprocessed emotions that got stuffed away today? Process whatever shows up in your inner world, perhaps with a relaxing activity or hobby. Spending time doing what you love is naturally leveling, restoring tranquility and balance to your emotional state.

I keep my mood in check by allowing the flow of life's emotional waves. I focus on joy to balance my mood and live in tranquility.

Restful Ritual

Tonight, take some time doing something you are good at—a hobby or other endeavor—to boost your endorphins as well as your self-esteem. You can help to balance your mood by doing something you love.

I FREE MY LIFE OF DRAMA AND NEGATIVITY.

Drama is a part of life, but inner peace is our preferred natural state. We all know that person who thrives on knowing everyone's business—the type that has a propensity for drama. Some of us have a subconscious enjoyment of chaos, even experiencing inner calm as an unfamiliar, unsafe burden. Living in habitual drama means living in constant stress—the central nervous system can never relax. Seeking drama can also be a form of self-protection, keeping you from feeling your emotions; by focusing on external theatrics, the internal landscape is ignored or suppressed. Like any addict, you may not realize you are self-medicating with drama. Detach from chaos and negativity and focus inward, choosing calm over calamity.

I remove myself from drama, gossip,
and negativity. I choose peace, love,
and stability as an act of self-care.

RESTFUL RITUAL

Do some self-reflection in your journal before bed. Do you gossip about others? Does this behavior really serve you? Consider making a pledge to yourself tonight to choose inner peace over gossip from now on.

242

My breath is my sanctuary.

When you think of the most peaceful person you know, what is it about them that makes them so calm? Do they have a daily routine that prioritizes their mental, physical, and spiritual well-being? The choices you make every moment impact your overall health. Mindful practices like simply focusing on the power of the moment and your breath connect you to calm. When we get anxious, we tend to hold our breath and forget to breathe. When navigating any moment of your life, choose to access a deeper sense of awareness by breathing in deeply and exhaling deeply. Know that this is always a safe place for you to return to—your breath is your sanctuary.

I relax into my sanctuary of self, letting go of external stimuli. I am calm and connected to my breath, knowing that all is well. I breathe deeply in and out as my resting state of mind.

Restful Ritual

Do a pursed-lip breathing exercise before bed, breathing in and out slowly and intentionally, with your lips pursed.

My body is my teacher.

When you feel overwhelmed, your body takes on the pressure to regulate your entire system, sometimes manifesting as pain. Though body pain can be tied to physical activity, aging, or lifestyle choices, it can also be tied to spiritual and emotional stress. Your body responds to how you feel and what you think. If you're stressed about a choice you need to make and suddenly stub your toe, it could be your body telling you to slow down and watch your next step. Energetically go into any body pain and listen to your body's messages there.

I connect with my body and ask what it needs. I listen to its guidance and honor this wisdom.

Restful Ritual

Go inward tonight with a foot soak. Put a few drops of lemongrass essential oil into a basin of warm water with a tablespoon of Epsom salt. While your feet soak, consider a choice you need to make. Where do you feel this indecision in your body? Give this area love as you consider the next steps toward making a decision.

I WITHDRAW FROM THE WORLD. I AM AT EASE.

The foundation for an excellent night's sleep begins with calming the mind and relaxing your mental landscape. When you go to bed each night, how does it feel in your mental space? Tonight, try getting out of your head as you hop into bed. The bedroom should be a sanctuary of safety and comfort. Instead of being trapped in your mind, escape through the physical presence of your body. Experience the art of simply being at ease in your own skin.

I focus less on the mental and more on the physical. I feel my body and the sensations on my skin. I lie in bed aware of my surroundings. My mind is open and calm, and my body is relaxed.

RESTFUL RITUAL

Change your bedding tonight; as you crawl into bed, feel the soft, fresh fabric wrap around you. Rest your head on your pillow and feel the support it gives you. How do your sheets feel against your skin? How does the comforter smell? Engage with all your senses.

The truth transmutes dark into light.

There are certain people in the world who take advantage of those around them, doing what they can to get what they want without ever giving in return. *This is not you.* You stand in your truth—you have love in your heart, show up with empathy, and dedicate yourself to helping others. If you've been harmed by people living from their shadow—people stunted by trauma, lacking empathy and self-awareness—remove yourself from the relationship. Invalidating, bullying behavior can only continue in the shadows; it cannot survive the light of truth and love. Don't let fear hide you from the world. Trust you are safe in your truth, protected by divine love and light.

I am not afraid of others' shadows—the light of my truth is a beacon of love and safety. I share it freely, without expecting anything in return.

Restful Ritual

Add an atmosphere of soft, inviting light to your bedroom through a small nightlight or Himalayan salt lamp, which is thought to purify the air and transmute darkness into light.

My breath is the medicine that heals my inner angst.

We live in a world where information comes at us from all angles. You may have intrusive thoughts too—thoughts that don't even feel like yours. It's draining to navigate this roller coaster of energy, and unhealed trauma makes it harder. We make ourselves so busy—overworking, overthinking, overconsuming—as an avoidance tactic, so we don't have to feel the aftereffects of the pain we have experienced. Healing is layered and takes time, but it doesn't have to be so difficult. Relax your central nervous system by breathing consciously throughout the day, reminding your body that it is safe.

I activate a new level of awareness by fueling my cells with oxygen. Mindful breathing cycles life through my entire being.

Restful Ritual

Make breath a priority tonight by considering the air quality in your bedroom—how can you make it better? One easy solution is to add a few plants, particularly snake or spider plants, both of which are known to be the most purifying, oxygen-producing plants.

I RELEASE MY PAST.
FORGIVENESS IS MY FREEDOM.

Do you turn into someone you don't recognize when you are around a certain person? The person who triggers you most could be a karmic connection, and these types of relationships can quickly turn toxic if you haven't learned the necessary lessons. A karmic relationship is fueled with intensity and challenges as a way for two souls to balance karma, address unhealed patterns, and grow. It can be addictive, feeling good at times, but once you do the inner work to heal your karmic patterns, the behaviors of a karmic connection will become unattractive to you. Forgive your past, learn the lessons, and set yourself free.

I close the karmic cycle. I am free
of past pain. No one can harm me
without my permission.

RESTFUL RITUAL

Do some karmic work before bed. Identify a troubled connection that you are ready to release. Visualize this person you want to release from your life is standing in front of you. Imagine a cord connecting the two of you from your cores, then take imaginary scissors and cut this cord. Feel the freedom as you release this attachment. And send the message, "Go your way, in peace, love, and harmony," as Dr. James Martin Peebles said.

3

Bedtime Mantras for Enjoying Dreams

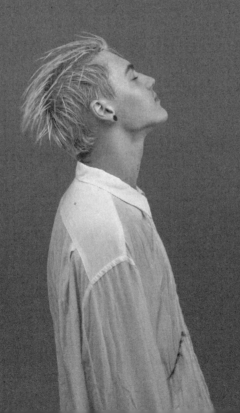

I'M IN FLOW STATE, WHERE WONDER ACTIVATES MY BODY.

Being Zen like the Buddha sounds nice in theory, but what if there really is an easy way to tap into this flow state? You *can* do this by harnessing the power of your alpha brain waves. Alpha waves create the calm, cool, collected state of mind that happens when you daydream, meditate, relax, or practice mindfulness. Setting the intention to induce this state is another way to achieve it. The next time you feel uneasy, shift your mood to an alpha-wave state by working with calm moon energy and an amethyst crystal. Amethyst is a healing stone that reduces anxiety and supports the body to achieve deeper sleep.

I relax my mind and body into a state of flow and ease. My cells are activated and alive with wonder.

REJUVENATION RITUAL

Invite the moon's energy to flow into your body tonight. Put a clean amethyst crystal into a glass of filtered water a few hours before bed, placing the glass in moonlight if possible. Drink mindfully before you go to sleep.

I AM ON A JOURNEY TO NIRVANA.

We live in such a fast-paced world; it's possible that your restless nights are due to this external influence. Everyone has different needs, in the same way that everyone is unique, and creating an effective nighttime routine for you involves understanding your needs—what is important and practical for you. Choose a mattress that works for your body, comfortable pillows that match how you sleep, and an environment that supports what you require for a good night's rest. Make sure you honor your needs and preferences when it comes to bedtime comfort—your personal sleep strategies create a stronger foundation for everything in your life. Recognize that your sleep is not an option but a daily necessity in your journey of self-discovery, self-awareness, and self-mastery.

The sleep solution for me is as unique as I am.
I honor my life's journey by honoring what I need
at night to obtain deep and peaceful rest.

REJUVENATION RITUAL

To induce deeper sleep, bring a fan or white-noise machine into your bedroom. (A white-noise sleep app is another option.)

I CAN ESCAPE FROM MY SELF-IMPOSED PRISONS.

Overthinking is one of the most counterproductive things, preventing us from feeling safe and calm, yet it is something we can easily fall into. If you've felt trapped in your head with obsessive thoughts, frequent rumination, and neurotic behavior, the solutions may seem as overwhelming as the overthinking itself! Instead of focusing on the discomfort, can you find the purpose—the lesson—behind it? Relax your mind by shifting your focus to honoring the situation and cultivating a sense of gratitude for the wisdom it offers. It's hard to see situations clearly when you are trapped in a fear vortex, but you can escape the pain by focusing on the positive.

I free myself from self-imposed mental angst by shifting from fear to curiosity. I change my mental landscape to look for the wisdom in all of my life's circumstances. Gratitude is my gatekeeper.

REJUVENATION RITUAL

Release yourself from anxious thoughts tonight by getting cozy under a weighted blanket, knowing you are safe and protected.

My frequency is vibrant and healthy.

If you've ever been in a great mood, then suddenly felt a huge dip for no tangible reason, it could be your vibrational energy. Managing your vibration means checking in on where your frequency is resonating and raising it as needed. Part of living a balanced life requires taking into account your vibrational health. Positive thoughts, healthy foods, daily movement, connecting with nature, and practicing mindfulness all keep your vibration high. Embracing colors is also a powerful way to stay vibrationally fit. Color therapy, also called chromotherapy, is the concept that colors impact our mood, improving mental and physical health. Bring more color into your life and watch how things transform for the better.

My vibrational health is sacred.
I honor my inner frequency by tuning in to
colors and higher vibrations.

REJUVENATION RITUAL

As you sit in bed tonight, look up hues of blue—do any resonate with you? Consider painting an accent wall that color or adding it to your bedding. Blue is recognized by the brain as mentally peaceful, evoking a state of calm.

Peace is my personal power, a gift from deep sleep.

When your brain overloads from overthinking, your cognitive function decreases and memory diminishes. Just like a computer maxed out on memory, your brain may start to run slower and stall. The same rules apply to the physical space of your bedroom. Clear out clutter, make sure it is dark enough, and minimize distractions (noise, screen time, etc.)—all practices of good sleep hygiene. When you mindfully care for your sleep space, you send the signal that this activity matters—that you care about and prioritize your sleep health as part of your overall well-being. Reclaim the personal power of inner peace by optimizing your sleep experience for a better night's rest.

I understand that rest is a great gift to myself, and I honor this fully. I love myself enough to foster peaceful sleep each night.

Rejuvenation Ritual

Tonight, take an inventory of your mood before bed—is it stressed or at peace? In what ways could you be more mindful about creating an atmosphere of peace to support more peaceful sleep?

I SURRENDER MY INSECURITIES TO THE STARS.

One of the biggest reasons we suffer in life is because we disrespect ourselves daily with self-doubt and self-judgment. When you invalidate your own experiences, your internal world can feel like a battlefield. Your immune system suffers, you have restless nights, and you become hypervigilant. But there is beauty in breakdown when you are open to seeing the opportunities available to you. One way to do this is to look up—to access the energy of the stars; you are made of the same components as they are. When self-doubt and insecurity get the best of you, lean on the stars to shine understanding on the shadows within. Your friends in the sky are always ready to lend support with their infinite light.

I acknowledge my doubt but don't let it stop me. The stars' guiding light washes away all fear and insecurity.

REJUVENATION RITUAL

Let yourself be the star that you truly are! Before bed tonight, have some fun painting your fingernails or toenails with glitter nail polish or use face or body glitter on your skin for fun.

I AM PROUD OF MY GROWTH.

Working on personal development, healing, and growing takes time and energy, but you are doing an amazing job! Doing this work can be challenging, especially when going through incredibly difficult changes in life. The key is to focus on stabilizing your energy by honoring your growth. Just like when a houseplant has outgrown its pot, with its roots all bunched up and tight, when you repot it in a bigger pot with fresh soil, it can take some time before the plant begins to thrive—the transition from the old to the new can be traumatic. Be patient with yourself and feel proud of how far you've already come.

My growing pains are grace in action.
I honor the path I am walking, for I am
expanding into new life experiences
that allow me to thrive.

REJUVENATION RITUAL

Give some care to a beloved houseplant tonight by repotting it. Move it into your bedroom for a comfortable climate as it transitions to its new home.

I ACCEPT WHAT I NEED OVER WHAT I WANT.

In life's transitional phases, moving from one chapter to the next can feel completely foreign and uncomfortable. When this happens, there may also be a grieving process. It is wise to think about your values and core needs during these times of transition. As you learn how to navigate the new aspects of your life—a process that may include letting go of a dream you were working toward—you can still be present for the new experiences and situations you find yourself in. Even when what you thought you wanted isn't what you needed, leading with your core needs will always make you feel more secure.

I don't force things to fit—what is meant for me will never pass me by. I surrender my will, release all expectations, and trust that I have what I need.

REJUVENATION RITUAL

Wind down the night with an online tai chi or qigong video. As you practice the gentle movements, focus on appreciation for all aspects of your life, especially the transition periods.

THE WISDOM WITHIN IS MY MENTOR.

Are you doing everything you can think of to figure out the best way forward in a challenging situation? Sometimes, we look to others for wisdom in cases like this. Maybe you are hiring coaches, taking online classes, or reading a lot of personal development books. While there's a time and place for accessing outside information, the best leaders and healers will always lead you back to your true self—what you need is already available *within you*. When you learn to trust the wisdom of personal experience, you expand into a greater depth of awareness and move forward in life with more grace. Take the path within to find the path without—this is the map to balance and wholeness.

My life experiences are my greatest teachers.
All the answers I seek are within.

REJUVENATION RITUAL

Put on a sleep mask and lie down in bed. Visualize a stressful situation in your life, then ask your inner wisdom how to solve it. Wash away your worries with the mask, feeling refreshed and at peace.

I HAVE THE POWER TO CHANGE THE COURSE OF MY LIFE.

If you feel like you don't have a choice in a situation, recognize that even this thought is a choice. Though it may feel like there is no opportunity to choose differently, it's often fear obscuring your options. We always have choices available to us; when we feel like we don't, we may be avoiding the potential outcomes. When necessary, the universe will come in and force change upon you, especially if you've been ignoring the signs. If this happens, trust the guidance you receive. Look at what you can control within the choices available to you. What option feels the most aligned with your true self? Balance your head and your heart, and you will always make the right choice.

I know I have many options available to me.
I approach these choices with an open mind
and heart—they never lead me astray.

REJUVENATION RITUAL

Keep your mind sharp and relaxed for decision-making by doing a crossword, sudoku, or word-find puzzle before bed.

I AM READY TO RECEIVE FULFILLMENT THROUGH MY DREAMS.

Fulfillment comes in many different forms, and often when we are doing what we love. Remember the last time you tapped into a skill, talent, or hobby and lost track of time? When you do what you love, contentment floods your entire being. This feel-good energy comes from aligning to your interests and values. When you live from your joy, you live a life of expansion. All of your dreams matter—the dreams and goals that you're working to achieve in your waking life and the dreams at night too. Let your dreams in the evening guide you to more clarity on how you can receive fulfillment in your waking life.

My dreams matter: they are the signature to my full potential. When I go to bed at night, I surrender, allowing my dreams in sleep to guide my dreams in waking life.

REJUVENATION RITUAL

Start to document the dreams you have in your journal. Make an intention tonight to remember and record your dreams in the morning.

I HAVE CONFIDENCE IN MYSELF AND MY DREAMS.

When you believe in yourself, you are a force to be reckoned with! But the opposite can have its own debilitating effects—when you don't believe in yourself, your visions may never actualize. The dreams you have in your heart are important, but you must take action to bring them to fruition, first by believing in your own power. Focus on your relationship with yourself to build up your confidence and courage—you've got this! Let go of any doubts and have some fun by tapping into the vast power of your internal dreamer.

When I focus on my dreams, I show the world that I matter—I believe in myself. I have all that I need to bring my ambitions to life.

REJUVENATION RITUAL

Tap into your inner source of abundance before bed. Lie down in your favorite spot in your home, place pyrite (a gold or green-colored crystal, great for attracting abundance) on your solar plexus chakra (the area of your diaphragm), and close your eyes. Radiate pride, self-confidence, and self-worth through the stone and your entire being.

I ALLOW MYSELF TO GRIEVE THE DREAM THAT DID NOT MANIFEST.

Some seasons of our life require us to be there for others more than ourselves. Maybe you had to give up a dream because you had to relocate to care for aging parents or sick children; an urgent project came up at work; or other outside demands impacted your life's direction. It's hard to move forward when you need to put others first, but you can restore balance by caring for yourself in small ways. Showing up for others is a part of your soul's expansive journey—a divine call to action. Trust that a deep lesson of love and greater understanding is in the making.

I am not off track or behind when I feel called to support others. I am gentle and patient with myself during these phases of my life.

REJUVENATION RITUAL

Infuse the peace and calm of bedtime into a worry stone or favorite crystal. Carry this stone or crystal in your pocket this week, releasing your worries every time you touch it.

I AM MINDFUL ABOUT THE CONTENT I CONSUME.

Your dreams at night can be a telling indicator of how your next day will go, and the same is true for nightmares. Have you ever had a bad dream that was so disturbing it stayed with you for days, or even months or years? Nightmares don't have to be feared; in fact, they contain valuable information that can help you navigate your waking life. You may be having nightmares because you've been experiencing anxiety and stress, or you're healing from trauma.[41] Maybe you can't stop listening to true-crime podcasts or doomscrolling on social media—if so, it could be keeping you up at night. Be more mindful of what you allow into your precious heart and headspace, especially before bed.

I am intentional about the information I consume and the choices I make. I remove myself from negative and fear-based energies, choosing to focus on calm instead.

REJUVENATION RITUAL

Start a seven-day digital content detox tonight, with no negative news, social media, or dramatic movies before bed. Commit to watching, reading, and listening to only calm, positive, or educational material.

I GIVE MY INNER CHILD LOVE AND DAILY CARE.

As we grow older, if we don't address painful experiences from the past, they negatively impact our thoughts, relationships, and careers—our overall quality of life. Seek to understand your inner child's needs to begin the healing process. This is not about blaming or sending negative thoughts to your parents or other caregivers; reclaiming your power and changing subconscious patterns means addressing your unmet needs from childhood—your inner child needs you. Take some time to get to know your young self, and embrace the honor of becoming the safe, loving space you've always wanted.

My inner child is part of me—we are one.
When I do the inner work to love and care for
this child, I heal us both.

REJUVENATION RITUAL

Prepare for bed by taking a bubble bath with a rubber duckie or other bath toy. As you sit in this carefree spirit of play, in your mind's eye, connect to a favorite childhood memory.

I GRACEFULLY GLIDE THROUGH ALL CHANGES IN MY LIFE.

Change happens to all of us, but do not despair. No matter what, you have grace as your navigator. Within all the choices you make, find inspiration in the joy and excitement for what is to come; replace all fear with love. When you do this, you feel more alive and secure. See the changes in your life as motivation to keep going—this life change is for your highest good! Through all of life's transitions, look to the future with trust and curiosity, carving each new path with openness and grace.

Change represents growth, and I welcome it. As the changemaker in my life and overseer of my destiny, I choose to navigate my journey with grace, joy, and love— my inner power.

REJUVENATION RITUAL

Enter dreamland early by lying down in bed with two cut slices of cucumber placed on your eyes. Get whisked away in your imagination by visualizing yourself on your dream vacation: Where are you, who are you with, and how are you enjoying yourself? You can even put aloe vera gel or water on your face for an added boost.

I RELEASE MY BURDENS TO MANIFEST MY HIGHEST TRUTH.

Manifesting new opportunities requires a willingness to make room for them. Letting go of the past may feel like you're giving up, but letting go is necessary to your soul's healing and expansion process. When you focus on something you desire, you're aligning to your truth in the present moment, which may involve aspects of yourself and your life that are no longer needed. These could be aspects of your character, relationships, or outdated ideas and beliefs. Like an animal who sheds its skin when it outgrows it, you are transitioning into a new phase of your life. Release yourself to enjoy the process and blessings to come.

I lay past burdens to rest and manifest from a place of love. I hold a vibration of truth for what I want, and my desires find their way to me.

REJUVENATION RITUAL

Before bed, brush your hair as a practice in letting go of the old. Focus on what you want to manifest, and close the practice with a blessing of love.

I AWAKE WITH CONFIDENCE AND CLARITY.

Do you have a nonnegotiable element in your sleep routine—something you must include to get a good night's sleep? Just like a child who needs their special teddy bear, these small rituals provide safety and comfort. Security in our evening routines also affects how we feel the next morning. The optimal goal when you follow your regular sleep routine is to rise feeling refreshed, but if you are not feeling as rested as you'd hoped and your days are harder to get through, consider revamping your bedtime routine. Has it turned boring or fallen out of sync with your needs? It's time to revise and refresh your must-have items and go-to habits at night to give your days a boost.

I prioritize my sleep routine to wake up refreshed each morning. The quality of my nights affects the quality of my days.

REJUVENATION RITUAL

Positive visualization can help you fall asleep. As you lay your head down tonight, close your eyes and envision a perfect day tomorrow. What does it look like?

My body deserves healthy nourishment and rest.

When is the last time you ate something because you were craving it and simply enjoyed it, 100 percent guilt free? In our society and many social circles, there tends to be a lot of pressure around food and eating habits: don't eat this, only eat that, eat at this time of day—all the rules and conflicting information get confusing. Social norms push popular diets and unreasonable beauty standards that just perpetuate self-criticism. When it comes to your health and the best diet for you, tune in to *your* body's clues and internal needs. Eat mindfully—what feels right for you and your body. Practice intuitive eating by listening to your body and following its messages.

I have a positive relationship with my body and food. I nourish my body with joy and ease, and I honor its needs daily.

Rejuvenation Ritual

Ask your body what it wants for a bedtime snack, then practice mindful eating. Use all of your senses to enjoy the food, giving thanks to it and your body.

I AM GRATEFUL FOR THE PEACE AND COMFORT OF MY BED.

When is the last time you thanked your bed, your pillows, your sheets, your blankets for supporting you every night? We don't usually give gratitude and empathy to objects, but everything is created with an energetic vibration attached to it—a life force is in all that exists. Think of every point on the supply chain that created your bedding, from the farmers who planted and picked the cotton to the fabric designers, the furniture makers, and the delivery drivers. Pay attention to your sleep environment by giving thanks to it. The more present you are in your bed, the more you can appreciate all it does for you.

When I am peaceful in my bed, I feel safe.
I appreciate this source of comfort and
all those who helped create this
experience for me.

REJUVENATION RITUAL

Tonight, pay homage to your bed. Share your experience of sleeping in it with the manufacturer of the matress or bedding by leaving an online review or sending a thank-you email.

Love is my guide—it never fails me.

When in the thick of life's challenges, people around you may try to offer comfort with comments like, "Think positive—it could be worse!" and "It can't be that bad!" Despite their good intentions, when life has knocked you to your knees, having hope can feel impossible. If you're in a similar place now and stuck in survival mode, trying to be positive is the last thing on your mind. To heal and move forward, a period of isolation and self-care may be needed—"time heals all wounds" when love leads the way. Perhaps it's time to seek professional help with a therapist, coach, trusted medical team, or support groups. Let your heart lead you forward to the care it requires.

Working through life's big challenges paves
my path to higher realms and perspectives.
I lean on love as my guide and strength.

Rejuvenation Ritual

Rest in an atmosphere of love tonight. Put several drops of jasmine essential oil (or your favorite scent) in a spray bottle of filtered water, and mist your pillows before bed.

I AM HONORED TO TAKE OWNERSHIP OF MY LIFE.

Pride is a tricky companion that gets in the way of patching up and maintaining beautiful connections. In twelve-step treatment programs, the eighth step involves determining who you've hurt in your past and taking responsibility—making amends. Take a look at your relationships and be honest with yourself: Who do you need to apologize to? Even if you didn't intend to cause pain, apologizing demonstrates love. (And by the way, saying "I'm sorry you feel that way" is not an apology!) Simply say "I'm sorry I made you feel this way" to take accountability and move on. Put yourself in other people's shoes, and make amends where needed.

I leave my pride behind and am honest in my relationships. I forgive myself for harming others, and I forgive others for harming me. Taking ownership sets me free.

REJUVENATION RITUAL

Tonight, as you wash your face before bed, thoughtfully repeat the words "I forgive myself for hurting [insert person's name]," and then "I forgive [insert person's name] for hurting me."

I PRIORITIZE A POSITIVE SLEEP ENVIRONMENT.

You may not be able to control your racing mind, but you can address the environment that you're sleeping in. Start by looking at the things around you that may be causing you to feel restless. This includes lighting, digital devices, sounds, even smells—anything distracting, annoying, or stressful that prevents you from focusing on a peaceful slumber. Creating a restful environment is the first way to address feeling calm and surrendered at night. When your thoughts are overactive from an overactive day, guiding them toward stillness through a positive sleep environment is something within your control.

I create calm through a peaceful environment.
The condition of my external world impacts
the condition of my internal world.

REJUVENATION RITUAL

Observe your bedroom from your bed—how does it make you feel? Is it calming or chaotic? When you're looking to create a perfect bedroom environment, go for cool, dark, and quiet. Consider one thing you can do for a better night's sleep tonight.

I RELEASE TENSION TO PREPARE FOR BED.

The aches and pains we experience physically are often tied to mental discomfort, like overthinking, chronic worry, and stress, creating a cycle of imbalance between the two. Instead of asking how you can have more energy in the day to push through this tension, consider listening to your body and resting instead. Shift your mindset to *My body is asking me to slow down and rest, and I honor its needs*. If you have nonstop fatigue in your body, take the time to focus on it with intention and moments of rest when your body needs it.

I release the tension tied to body and thought imbalances from an overburdened day. I listen to and honor my body's need for stillness and rest.

REJUVENATION RITUAL

Do a body scan in bed before falling asleep, paying attention to how you feel and where. Visualize a warm golden light spreading serenity throughout your whole body, releasing tension and discomfort along the way.

I AM ACTUALIZED BY LOVE AND THE UNFOLDING JOURNEY.

Did you ever sit in a friend's new car, then suddenly, you wanted a new car? There are times when we desire things because we believe that having them will make us happier than we are now. But we didn't know we wanted it until we saw it. Sometimes seeing is believing, other times we must believe in order to see. No matter what, recognize that your dreams and goals coming true does not necessarily guarantee happiness, nor does it define you as a person. When you chase your dreams from a place of *I need this, so others will see what I have*, ego and fear are making choices based on low self-worth. Focus on manifesting your dreams from a place of love, releasing your attachment to the outcome. The journey to manifest your goal is the true reward.

I am actualized each day as I show up from a place of love. This is my true purpose and the measure of a life well lived.

REJUVENATION RITUAL

With a rose quartz crystal in your hands and love in your heart, prepare for lucid dreaming by meditating intentionally on what you want to dream about tonight.

MY SAFETY COMES FROM WITHIN.

Are you always on the lookout for what could go wrong, seeing the world as a risky place? If your mind is pre-occupied by worst-case scenarios, you are on high alert unnecessarily. Maybe you've learned through personal experience that you can't always rely on others—people can let you down. This burden feels heavy, weighing on your soul. Because of this clouded lens, you're understand-ably hesitant to take risks, but you're also missing beneficial opportunities. Wanting security is wise, but be careful that you're not confusing protection with unchecked fear. Often, the best things for your life's growth is just outside your comfort zone.

I feel comfortable in the uncomfortable aspects of life. I am safe in all situations because my safety is forever present, coming from within.

REJUVENATION RITUAL

Before bed, create a safe escape in your mind. Think about all the visceral details, like the colors, smells, and textures of this place. Feel your body there, and focus on how calm it makes you feel.

My boundaries are a beautiful extension of self-respect.

Personal boundaries are vital for healthy, secure relationships, but they can be hard to establish. From a young age, we are conditioned to conform to the world around us, even if it goes against our personal perspectives and space. Setting personal boundaries in adulthood is about safety and the lines we draw to honor our comfort level in relation to others. If you're a people pleaser or empath, you may not even know what your boundaries are. If saying no to someone makes you uncomfortable, there's a learning curve ahead, but you can start small. Much like a child learning to walk, protecting your sovereignty takes practice. Start by protecting yourself with clear communication on what your boundaries are.

My personal boundaries represent
self-respect, self-loyalty, and self-love.
I deserve to feel safe in the world.

Rejuvenation Ritual

Practice feeling your personal boundaries by tapping, pressing, or squeezing different places of your body. This is a wonderful somatic way to recognize your boundaries and get in touch with your body's needs. Commit to addressing one boundary infringement this week.

The night sky illuminates my deepest desires.

Burnout is a state of mental and physical exhaustion that can quickly turn into a lack of self-connection and decreased self-fulfillment. When you're burnt out, it's impossible to focus on your dreams, yet having dreams is the signature foundation of a fulfilling life. This is why it's so important to balance daily demands—to prevent burnout. What is your golden dream—the deepest desire you have yet to actualize? Give yourself permission to trust your desires, and dive right into their manifestation. Don't let the distraction of daily demands dim the light of what you truly want. Your potential is as endless as the night sky above.

My dreams outshine daily demands and social pressures. I choose to focus on my heart's desires as often as I can.

Rejuvenation Ritual

Tonight, look out your window or go outside to find a star to wish upon. As you do, let this be a declaration of your truest desire. Allow the stars to be your guide.

I WELCOME NEW OPPORTUNITIES WITH COURAGE AND ENTHUSIASM.

Building a bright future does not have to be a distant dream; every move you make today—every thought, every interaction, every effort—is either contributing to or deterring from the vision of your ideal life. When you are working toward a goal and don't see results, it can become discouraging. This is the moment when you might succumb to doubt and fear and give up on your dream, but this is the precise moment you must keep going! Making your dreams come true is not about the outcome but a lifestyle of manifestation. Bravely show up every day and be ready to play, exploring your world and all the opportunities available to you.

I take proactive steps daily to focus on my vision and activate my dreams. I commit to my heart's desires and joyfully welcome the expansive journey.

REJUVENATION RITUAL

Tonight, usher in new beginnings by replacing screen time with family time. Make a plan to spend time this week in the company of people you love.

My dreams are healing and expansive.

In a REM state, your dreams take you deep into your unconscious mind, to worlds of new perspectives and opportunities. In addition to expanding your heart and mind, this deep sleep gives your cells time to heal and replenish. Set the intention to remember your dreams at night, incorporating their messages as part your healing journey. Likewise, the dreams you have in your waking life expand your soul and heal your heart. When you go for what you want, you resonate with possibility. Don't be afraid to dream bigger and brighter! Your light shines on the unknown to blaze the path forward into creation.

My dreams open new doors and illuminate things I could not conceive of before. I prioritize my sleep to access my dreams for healing and manifestation.

REJUVENATION RITUAL

Invite illumination and healing into tonight's bedtime routine. Light a candle and gaze into the flame, setting the intention to remember your dreams and record their insights in your journal in the morning.

My intuition makes me stronger.

Access to the five physical senses (touch, taste, sight, smell, hearing) is not something everybody has. Some are born without it or lose their senses through accidents, disease, aging, etc. For most of us, using our senses is something we don't think much about—that is, until we lose one. After that, we rely on other senses to fill in for what is lost. Your inner vision, often called clairvoyance, is an intuitive language that senses energy—images in the mind's eye or external auras. Everyone has access to intuition, even if they are physically blind. This inner seeing provides strength and stability in all areas of your life.

I honor the visions of my soul—my intuition.
I see clearly what is ahead of me and for
my highest good.

Rejuvenation Ritual

Tonight, consider getting an intuition buddy, and reach out to see if they are receptive to exploring energy experiences together. Set up a meeting this week, perhaps starting with analyzing a dream you each had recently.

I CHOOSE EMPOWERING BELIEFS TO SHAPE MY REALITY.

When is the last time you took a stroll down memory lane with gratitude and joy versus judgment and regret? Our lives are made up of many moments strung together, and the ways we reflect on these experiences shape our perspective on life. You may clump your experiences in a manner that creates a limiting belief, such as, *I was bullied as a child, so I am an easy target.* The opposite could be, *I was bullied as a child, and it made me stronger.* When you reflect on your life, string together its moments with empowerment, releasing any old beliefs that hinder you.

I've lived an amazing life and celebrate my journey so far. I choose empowering thoughts to experience all life has to offer me.

REJUVENATION RITUAL

Look at a photo of you before age ten to access your inner child before bed. Send loving thoughts to little you as you think about a positive childhood memory. (If you struggle to find one, imagine a positive experience you wish you'd had.)

I EXPLORE LIFE'S CONTRAST, IT BRINGS CLARITY AND HEALING.

We live in a world of illusions, fear-based agendas, and deception, but we also live in an honest, compassionate, loving world—both coexist; we can't have one without the other. Darkness and light, deception and love—two opposite sides of the same coin. To be on Earth is to explore this contrast; it brings clarity to what matters to you. The law of polarity says that everything in life has an opposite. If you're experiencing a difficult situation such as a layoff, divorce, or health issues, tune in to the opposite—your dream job, a happy relationship, a healthy body—for a new perspective. It is here where the lesson and wisdom reside.

I honor the law of polarity in the world and seek its balance. I actively pursue the entire truth for optimal healing and growth.

REJUVENATION RITUAL

Explore the law of polarity in your journal before bed, applying it to a troubling situation in your life. List the negative aspects, then list their opposites. What wisdom does this reveal?

I STEP OUT OF MY COMFORT ZONE TO FEEL ALIVE.

Living a vibrant life requires giving yourself permission to feel the energy of being in your body fully, no matter what. Allow yourself to go for opportunities that push your boundaries but bring you joy. Feeling the passion, excitement, and adrenaline of doing something new and exciting supports a balanced life. Getting out of your comfort zone is one of the fastest ways to stretch and rejuvenate all areas of your life. Get out of your own way by trying something new. Be brave—you've got this! You'll be surprised by how alive and energized you feel.

I feel alive when I challenge myself to do new things. I get out of my comfort zone to access a deeper sense of self and vitality.

REJUVENATION RITUAL

Practice sitting with your dislikes in your journal tonight. Is there something you disliked as a kid but haven't touched since childhood? Try it this week and see if your opinion has changed.

I UPHOLD MY STANDARDS DESPITE THE EXPECTATIONS OF OTHERS.

The stress and burnout that so many people feel is shared—we relate to one another through our stress points. Take an inventory of the people around you. Are they stressed out and prone to complaining? Do they drain you? If so, they could have an addiction to stress, and you may be supporting those codependent patterns. Ask yourself: *Is the stress I feel a way to relate to them or is this stress my own?* You have your own journey to manage without having to carry other people's burdens too. Tonight, release this responsibility, and let your mind and spirit rest.

I will not let burnout, stress, or overwhelm
be a way in which I relate to others.
The less I stress, the more I rest.

REJUVENATION RITUAL

Tonight, consider a partnership of mutual benefit. Do you have a friend who may need support and is also a good cheerleader? Ask them this week if they'd like to be a support buddy as you both work to destress and recalibrate.

I AM READY TO RECEIVE THE ABUNDANCE OF MY DREAMS MANIFESTED.

You've turned a major corner in your life and a new era is upon you. The dreams you have at night give clues to the next inspired action—a secret language of signs, symbols, and concepts about possible directions you're going in your waking life. Allow your dreams to be part of your personal guidance system as you enter into a new layer of your life. You can also engage with the energy of moonstone to support your unfolding dreams. Work with your unconscious mind to create these new realities.

I welcome abundance and embrace the richness of life. My dreams lead me to a joyful existence.

REJUVENATION RITUAL

As you fall asleep tonight, set the intention to receive guidance in your dreams and enhance them with moonstone energy. The element of water rules moonstone, so charge your stone by holding it under tap water for a few minutes. Place it under your pillow to welcome in your new era of abundance.

I CELEBRATE EVERY EMOTIONAL EXPERIENCE WITH JOY.

Your mind can focus on happiness and disappointment, excitement and rejection, victory and loss simultaneously. For example, if you think about a favorite memory from childhood, you can probably recall the same experience having multiple emotions tied to it, not just the pleasant ones. Consider that your emotions are not good or bad and that your experiences don't need to be qualified this way either. Tonight, as you wind down, celebrate your life so far, *exactly as it is*. Instead of judging your disappointments and losses, give them credit for their lessons. Focus on these, too, as victories to cultivate a joyful frame of mind, no matter what, every night before you go to bed.

I feel better when I focus on the positive outcomes of every life circumstance. Each day is special, and I celebrate its wins.

REJUVENATION RITUAL

Before bed, jot down three things that went well today in your journal. Be as specific as you can and then give yourself a high five!

I FOSTER INNER TRANQUILITY BY LISTENING TO SILENCE.

Where in your life have you been distracted? We spend so much time in our waking life trying to achieve things. Whether it is an exercise goal, relationship, job title, or performance award, it is exhausting to force our way through life. We sometimes don't even realize how distracting the little things are in our environment, like noise. Sirens, the neighbor's barking dogs, your kids, the TV—how can you possibly be productive or calm with so much audible chaos? Research shows that white noise can save your sleep, and it's perfect for masking loud disruptions.[42] Commit to addressing your home's noise pollution to create a more tranquil sleep environment.

I choose ease and calm in my evening environment, supporting inner tranquility by softening external distractions.

REJUVENATION RITUAL

Discover peace and quiet tonight through a sound detox! If you cannot eliminate the noise pollution in your surroundings, turn on a fan or white-noise playlist (online), or consider purchasing a white-noise machine or app.

Acceptance and love fuel my lifelong evolution.

When going through a spiritual awakening, your perspective widens and your awareness deepens. But what many of us don't realize is that this happens again and again in life—you are always evolving to reach new layers of yourself. The greatest gift you can give to this process and to others is to heal. When you heal wounded patterns, you transform relationships, improve your self-image, and repair your family lineage, providing future generations with a new foundation for relating to others—one grounded in wholeness and love. Tonight, be thankful for your healing process and lifelong evolution.

When I focus on my healing, I give power to awakening and expansion—the greatest gift I give to myself and others. This labor of love and acceptance is my legacy.

Rejuvenation Ritual

Tonight, create a small altar in your home with photos and items that remind you of your ancestors. Ask them for their wisdom and their support on your healing path.

I LOVINGLY SET FREE THE THOUGHTS THAT DON'T SERVE ME.

Not every thought requires attention. The ego mind, for example, is judgmental, competitive, fear based, and extremely protective; it can take your thoughts and you into a negative tailspin. But your true self—the spiritual self— knows when thoughts are based on illusions and fear.

Choose your thoughts the same way you choose an outfit to wear: Do you want to feel confident and functional today or worried and uncomfortable? Inspired thoughts easily outweigh the ego's when you experience the love and joy they produce. Making choices in life with clarity and positivity aligns you with opportunities. Free yourself from the confinement of fear-based thoughts by lovingly letting them go.

Each thought is an opportunity to build and grow or reflect and release. I set free those thoughts that do not serve me to make room for opportunities that do.

REJUVENATION RITUAL

Reflect and release in your journal before bed. Jot down some of the limiting thoughts from your day—use the moonlight and/or night sky to acknowledge them, and then release them with love.

I ACKNOWLEDGE MY LIMITATIONS TO GROW PAST THEM.

We get indoctrinated into belief and behavioral systems based on the culture we're born into. Socio-economic factors, environment, gender, and race all impact your life's blueprint. In psychology, the term *cognitive bias* refers to how a person's learned beliefs, opinions, and attitudes—aspects they may not even be aware of—inform how they process information.[43] Life gets filtered through a clouded lens, distorting your thinking and impacting every area. Gender bias, ageism, politics, and more can negatively impact your view of others. Remember, every person is a unique individual. If you label people based on false belief, you limit your humanity. Tonight, be more aware of your own perspectives and the way they serve or hinder you.

I see all people free of judgment, the way I want them to see me. I take accountability for my perspective and how it plays a role in my interactions.

REJUVENATION RITUAL

Commit yourself tonight to personal accountability. Reach out to someone you've hurt, even if unintentionally, and make it right. Speak from your heart and apologize.

I AM GRATEFUL FOR EVERY PART OF MY LIFE.

Your life is a living manifestation of your dreams. However, it's challenging to appreciate the things that are going well if you still have unresolved childhood trauma or issues. These past pains don't go away when you grow up; they stow away, restricting your movement and freedom until they're properly addressed. Fortunately, in adulthood, you can be the person you needed when you were younger. Start with gratitude, appreciating all that you've been through *and survived*, especially the difficult parts. Accept how your life has played out so far and send love to heal what is wounded. This is gratitude for a life well lived.

My life is an unfolding, creative, rewarding adventure. I do not attach myself to any outcome or experience. I am grateful for every day.

REJUVENATION RITUAL

Comfort your inner child as you snuggle into bed. What aspect of your childhood are you most grateful for? Spend time visualizing this tonight as you go to sleep. You can even look at a photo of little you and hug it as you drift off to dreamland.

I EMBRACE SMALL CHANGES TO MANIFEST BIG RESULTS.

What helps you feel good is perhaps different from the other people in your household, but the common thread is that you all do the best you can to feel better. Even with others around you, you can implement small changes that make profound differences to your ability to thrive. Focus on something that is important to you, such as feeling stronger, and then prioritize a routine to meet this need. It starts with the choices you make when you first wake up and every choice after that, even up to bedtime; aligning with your intention will ultimately manifest it.

*I make small changes in my daily
routines that align with my bigger goals.
Manifestation is built on every choice I make,
from morning to night.*

REJUVENATION RITUAL

Studies show that physical activity can help to reduce sleep disorders, such as insomnia, daytime sleepiness, and sleep apnea.[44] Set time aside tonight to create a sleep-friendly exercise routine that you can stick to over the next month. Stretching, yoga poses, tai-chi, whole-body vibrating machines,[45] or a gentle moonlight walk with your pet are good options.

MY NIGHTMARES OFFER INSIGHTS TO MY REALITY.

Just like making fear-based choices can turn into nightmares during waking life, stress and worries can manifest in your dreams as nightmares. Remember that nightmares are not your reality, but they do provide clues of your fears in your waking life. The next time you have a nightmare, look at the attributes of the dream: What was it that frightened you (a person, the circumstances, etc.)? Why was it a nightmare? One person's nightmare is not necessarily another's. Realize your nightmares are not happening to harm but to guide you. Though it may not be immediately evident, your nightmares offer a well of assistance intended just for you.

I solve problems in my waking life by understanding what scares me in my dreams. Identifying my fears leads to healing and resolve.

REJUVENATION RITUAL

Listen to calming music before bed, allowing its energy to soothe you into a positive sleep experience. As you fall asleep soundly, open yourself to receiving your dreams' wisdom and messages without fear.

LOVE IS MY NATURE.

Love is like a flashlight, illuminating the way forward in the darkness. When you are going through a difficult time, you may not know how you're going to make it through, but you can always find purpose in your pain. Trust that you will not only make it but that you will come out stronger and wiser than before. To support your body and self-regulation in times of uncertainty, tune in to your body's circadian rhythm. Keeping a consistent sleep schedule is one of the best things you can do to maintain a healthy circadian rhythm and feel balanced.[46] When you lead with love, you lead with faith in yourself, and this self-determination is a powerful force.

I choose to remain optimistic through life difficulties. I open up to the light, guidance, and love of my true nature.

REJUVENATION RITUAL

Depending on your wake-up schedule, consider opening your curtains before bed to allow yourself to regulate your circadian rhythm by waking with the sun. You could also investigate using a sunrise alarm clock.

I HAVE ALL THE SUPPORT
I NEED.

There are lessons that your soul came here to learn, and you can never be in the wrong place at the wrong time; the opportunity for growth is always available to you. Keep your mind and heart open, and the answers will come as signs, synchronicities, and well-timed support. Ask the Universe for help, pray to your higher power, and focus on the answers you receive. Your dreams offer guidance too; consider them to be the words of a wise counselor. And remember to lean on your guides for support through your process. All of these tools offer higher perspective, purpose, and motivation on your sacred life's journey.

Learning and growing is my soul's sacred purpose. I expand into higher vibrations with the loving energy and guidance of the universe, my spirit helpers, and my dreams.

REJUVENATION RITUAL

Write a presleep poem or prayer that invites the support of your spiritual helpers. Ask for this guidance to also appear in your dreams.

Even after the darkest nights, I rise.

Does it feel like the deadline is fast approaching? It's easy to feel trapped and without options when the pressure's on, let alone being able to relax and appreciate anything. Sometimes, the only way to make it out of a tough situation is to go straight through it—*keep going!* Make one choice at a time, and dive deeper into the dark—it's the only way to reach the light of a new day. Do your best to avoid overwhelm by breathing deeply and keeping a steady pace. The call of daily demands is persistent, but it does eventually quiet. Release the troubles you experienced today and welcome the peace of the night. This, too, shall pass.

I have patience, grace, and self-compassion in difficult times. I always rise.

Rejuvenation Ritual

Dab a few drops of valerian root oil (nature's herbal valium) onto the back of your neck or the bottoms of your feet to relax and fall asleep more easily.[47] An alternative is drinking a nighttime tea, which often contains valerian root.

I TREAT MYSELF WITH LOVE AND RESPECT.

Self-love isn't just about spa days, bubble baths, pedicures, or mud masks; true self-love is about understanding your value and living in ways that reflect this. It comes from a place of self-respect. The more you love yourself, the more you understand yourself; through self-understanding, you show up in the world with more loving awareness, compassion, and acceptance. You don't take things so personally, and you forgive easily. Practice self-love through the art of nonattachment. Start by removing unhealthy behaviors and limiting thoughts that are rooted in self-judgment or shame; you deserve to feel accepted and worthy.

Self-love is my compass, and I choose me every day. I love myself exactly the way that I am.

REJUVENATION RITUAL

Tonight, stand in front of a mirror and look at a part of your body that is different than it used to be. Reflect on what life event resulted in the change (having children, an injury, getting older, stress, etc.). Honor this part of you by giving thanks for this beloved part and this beloved *you*.

I REMOVE MY MASK AND CHOOSE AUTHENTICITY.

Being vulnerable around others is an opportunity to share your inner world with the outer world—a beautiful way to build deeper connections. The next time a friend asks you how you are, instead of responding automatically with "I'm good," be honest. Maybe you're having a hard day—share that openly with them; let others see your true experiences of life. As you allow yourself to be more vulnerable, you enhance the connection with yourself too: you no longer wear a mask or hide behind fear. This authenticity brings you closer to those who truly value, respect, and support you— relationships based on a lasting foundation of love.

When I share my feelings with others,
it is a gift to myself. I value real,
lasting connections grounded in
authenticity and love.

REJUVENATION RITUAL

In your journal tonight, draw a picture of the mask you wear— what fears does it protect? Think about how you want to address these fears to show up more authentically moving forward.

My commitment to my happiness opens new doors.

Do you ever ask yourself, *Is this the life I really want?* Maybe you keep daydreaming about going a completely different direction, such as living abroad and eating pastries in Portugal, or turning your passion into a career, or adopting your first child in your fifties. Reinventing yourself can be a terrifying yet empowering part of your life journey, especially when you allow yourself to grow into who you truly are. As you tap deeper into your values, you learn more about yourself; you release what doesn't serve you and naturally evolve. The key is to not resist these urges. Grow with the energy of your desires, and realize it is always okay to follow your heart.

I choose myself and my joy when I honor my heart's calling. It's never too late to change directions.

Rejuvenation Ritual

Clean your bathroom mirror before bed, holding the intention to wash away all fear and blocks that are holding you back. Fall asleep peacefully, knowing you've washed away the blocks preventing you from embracing your true self and your dreams.

I HARNESS THE POTENTIAL OF MY SUBCONSCIOUS MIND TO CREATE MY IDEAL REALITY.

Have you ever been asleep and questioned yourself or the circumstances in a dream, then made a conscious choice to redirect the dream's outcome? This is essentially a lucid dream—you're asleep but aware that you're dreaming. You can practice lucid dreaming by setting the intention before bed to recognize when you are in a dream state. Not only will you feel more in control, but you will deepen the connection with yourself. It is empowering to be the director of your own creative adventure. And when you align to your dreams in sleep, it's easier to manifest your wildest dreams in life.

I dive deep into my unconsciousness to access its fullest potential. I create my reality by focusing on the manifestation of my ideal life.

REJUVENATION RITUAL

Prepare for lucid dreaming tonight. As you drift off to sleep, recall a recent dream that you'd like to revisit, then set this simple intention: *I will know I am dreaming tonight.*

I SEE MY TRUE WORTH AND HONOR IT FULLY.

Wanting attention from others is human nature, but if you grew up in an environment where your emotional or physical needs weren't met due to neglectful, abusive, or absent caregivers, you probably equated love to performing, thinking, *I must please, do, fix, help to be loved.* This broken belief system can lead to people pleasing; dysfunctional, toxic, co-dependent relationships; trauma bonds; and self-sabotaging. Outsourcing your worth to the validation of others is a core childhood wound that takes time and effort to heal. Fortunately, with gentle kindness and intentional loving awareness, you can begin to mother yourself back to the wholeness of your already beautiful being.

My worth is not dependent on anything outside of me—I validate myself from within. I honor myself exactly as I am with respect, love, and care.

REJUVENATION RITUAL

Practice validating yourself in your journal before bed. Write three things that you value most about yourself and your life's decisions, and offer love and gratitude for each one.

I HOLD THE POWER TO TURN MY DREAMS INTO REALITY.

Sometimes we hide behind our to-do lists to avoid going after our dreams. If we don't follow through, then we won't be disappointed, right? If we don't act, an era of mystery lives on—the true work to maintain the dream remains unknown. A fantasy, after all, still promises potential but nothing that can really hurt us. When you take action on your visions, you move from being an observer of your life experience to being its creator, and being the creator means *you* have all the power! Tap into this power and take inspired action to do the work and see your vision through to reality. Your dream and its rewards are worth it.

My dreams are my legacy of a life fulfilled.
I do the work so I can enjoy the rewards.

REJUVENATION RITUAL

Focus inward by working with a mandala tonight. Draw or print one out and color it in, which can reduce anxiety.[48] As you color, focus on your ideal life in your mind's eye, believing it is possible.

I RESPECT OTHERS THE SAME WAY I WISH TO BE RESPECTED.

Learning about personality disorders and mental health conditions helps to understand relationship dynamics and yourself better. For example, "dark triad" traits involve unpredictability, lack of empathy, and seeing people as a means to an end; opposite these are the "light triad" traits, which involve a belief that humans are good individually and collectively, and that all beings should be treated as an end in and of themselves.[49] Which traits do you relate to? Not everyone sees the world the way you do, and one way isn't necessarily better than another. Make sure you are respecting others in the same way you wish for them to respect you.

I do my part and show loving kindness to all, including myself. I respect others to foster the same in return.

REJUVENATION RITUAL

Do some soul searching in your journal before bed. Look at your standards for yourself and what you're tolerating from others. Make a list of the things you're settling for and what they are costing you, then commit to reversing this trend.

I AM WORTHY OF MY DESIRES.

Your dreams are indicators of what is truly important to you. You have a value system that you align to, and the goals you feel in your heart are manifestations of these driving needs. But when your actions don't align with your words, you are out of integrity with yourself. You're most likely operating from a place of low self-respect and worth. If you're struggling to feel worthy of your desires, it will be apparent in your actions. You may neglect taking care of yourself or settle for unsatisfying life conditions that don't fulfill you. Instead of ignoring your own desires, focus on the root issue—the feeling of not being good enough. Start by creating an intentional self-love practice that prioritizes self-care and positive thinking.

I focus on my worth by taking care of myself daily. I manifest my dreams into reality with self-love.

REJUVENATION RITUAL

Listen to a sound-healing meditation tonight with a focus on what self-doubt is trying to tell you. What do you need to manifest your heart's desires?

WHAT IS MEANT FOR ME COMES TO ME WITH EASE.

We all want something that we don't have, and the more you focus on how you don't have it, the more it falls away. In manifesting, you can't get what you want when you're focusing on how it's not here. Tonight, recognize that what you desire desires you too—it's on its way. The form and timing may differ from what you expect, so relax and enjoy the journey. All is in right order. Taking care of yourself is an important aspect of manifesting your desires, so relax into the evening and trust in divine timing.

The universe is abundant and gives me what is meant for me. I align with opportunities that align with this purpose.

REJUVENATION RITUAL

The art of preparing your evening tea is a wonderful opportunity to connect with the present moment. Grab your favorite teacup, leave your phone in the other room, and sip your tea in silence as you focus on what you want. Imagine it coming to you with ease and joy; allow this vision to warm your heart.

I BRAVELY ASK FOR HELP WHEN I NEED IT.

Learning how to receive is one of the greatest gifts you can give yourself. If you've spent most of your life showing up for others and taking care of them, tonight is a reminder that you need care too. Caregivers need care, healers need healing, and supporters need support—all roles experience this need. If you are a natural giver, giving to yourself may require a simple change in perspective: the art of receiving enhances the art of giving. Identify a need of yours, send a prayer to the universe for assistance, and fall asleep in peace as you open yourself to receiving it.

I honor my giving nature by allowing myself to receive. The best way to love others is to love myself.

REJUVENATION RITUAL

Mix a few drops of lavender essential oil and coconut oil, and put it behind your ears and on your forehead. As you drift off to sleep, present a need to your guides (higher self, God, the universe), then release the request to their loving care.

I ATTRACT GENUINE AND TRUSTWORTHY PEOPLE.

There is a difference between right and *sort-of* right. Doing the right thing even when no one is watching is acting with integrity. But some people, if given the chance, might see what they can get away with, acting from fear, egoism, or self-preservation. We either make head-based choices (analytical and rational) or we make heart-based choices (empathic and centered in our feelings), and discernment is the marriage of the two. Being able to recognize when something feels right or wrong is the sixth-sense muscle you can buff up daily. When you meet new people, pay attention to both your mind and your body awareness. Maybe you feel uneasy or peace, or maybe you hear something that feels off. Trust your discernment to guide you toward sound decisions.

I am always protected with divine love.
I attract kind and trustworthy people
with its guidance.

REJUVENATION RITUAL

Put on your favorite sleep mask, close your eyes, and identify all the ways in which you trust yourself. Celebrate the genuine aspects of your character, and tap into the love you feel in your heart.

308

I TREAT MYSELF LIKE SOMEONE I ADORE.

Every situation in your life is an opportunity to monitor your self-image. If you're in a situation that feels unjust, instead of pointing the finger at the other person who is not treating you with the respect you deserve, ask yourself if *you* are treating yourself with this respect. Why are you staying in disrespectful situations? Check in with this simple question: *Am I treating myself like someone I adore?* If you're staying in a situation and hoping it will get better, you're giving away the value of your true worth. Be honest with yourself about who you spend your time with and how you spend your days. Surround yourself with people who respect and value you as well as themselves.

I adore and love myself in everything I do.
I am an example of self-respect and kindness.

REJUVENATION RITUAL

Before bed, draw a warm bath and add your favorite bath oil. Use a loofah or wash cloth and massage your body in a circular motion, honoring the gorgeous soul that you are.

I HONOR MY EMPATHIC NATURE.

If you've ever been told you're too sensitive, or if you can't help but feel the emotions of others, you could be an empath. Empaths are attuned to others' emotional experiences. If you're an empath or highly sensitive person (HSP), you may think you are somehow damaged. But you're not the odd duck after all—actually, 15 to 20 percent of the population is an HSP.[50] Don't ever underestimate the power of your empathic nature; your ability to hold space for others helps those around you. However, burnout is a common challenge for empaths, so make sure you have a good work–life balance by upholding your boundaries and getting plenty of self-care.

I embrace my sensitivity, using my empathy to support others and myself. I trust my emotions to connect deeper with all of life.

REJUVENATION RITUAL

Before sleep, sit on the edge of your bed and close your eyes, turning your hands face down and visualizing your energy moving down to the earth. This is a simple way of grounding yourself for stress relief and optimal rest.

I RETREAT INWARD FOR DIVINE INSPIRATION.

When the world is gnawing at you for attention, you don't have to succumb to the pressure; in fact, you can tune it all out. When you sleep, your body goes into a cozy cocoon mode, tuning out the world completely, and your dreams are a reprieve from daily demands. Pay more attention to your sleep health, because the quality of your nightly routine and dreams offers the beautiful gift of rest and relaxation. Your mind and consciousness go into deeper realms as you detach from the rest of the world. Reclaim the personal power of divine inspiration through the quality of your sleep and dreams at night.

I consciously release my daily burdens by relaxing my mind and body. My dreams take me to places of joy and wonder as I sleep.

REJUVENATION RITUAL

Spend some time alone before bed, reflecting on a time when you listened to your intuition and a time when you did not. How do these decisions feel different? Attune to the energy of intuition to tap into divinity tonight.

I AM MY GREATEST INVESTMENT.

It's time to treat yourself better. The first step to understanding your self-worth is to acknowledge it. When is the last time you really stopped and gave yourself kudos for all your skills, talents, and experiences? Do you recognize how you're positively contributing to the world? Most of us don't think about what makes us unique; we compare ourselves to others instead, focusing on achievements and measuring up to outside standards. But you're a gift to this world just by being who you are *right now*. Investing in yourself demonstrates faith in this worth and value. When you understand what you bring to the table, you're more likely to meet others who appreciate and respect you in kind.

I understand my worth and know my value.
I invest in myself as the most valuable asset
I have to offer the world.

REJUVENATION RITUAL

Start planning tonight for a date with yourself this week. Go shopping for a small gift, eat brunch at your favorite café, take yourself to a movie—whatever sounds carefree and fun!

THE CELLS IN MY BODY VIBRATE IN PERFECT HARMONY.

Have you ever wondered why breathwork or meditation is so relaxing? It has a lot to do with activating your vagus nerve. The vagus nerve is the core communication channel connecting your brain to automatic functions like breathing and digestion; it is also responsible for calming the fight-or-flight response, because when it is activated, it signals to your body you are safe, that no threat is around. It means you have a healthy responses to stress.[51] When you deal with chronic stress, however, your brain never gets the memo—you stay stuck in overdrive. No wonder we're all exhausted! The good news is you can strengthen your vagus nerve like you would your muscles at the gym. Throughout the day, even when you are not stressed, calming your breath and body stimulates the vagus nerve, bringing your intention back to balance.

Peace and calm are my ideal state. When I am in harmony, my cells live there too.

REJUVENATION RITUAL
Your vagus nerve loves calm as much as quality sleep! Listen to meditative music or an audiobook narrated by someone with a calming voice to usher yourself into peaceful rest tonight.

I AM ALIVE, WELL, AND THRIVING.

Pay attention to what makes you feel alive—the elements of life that inspire you and burn with the desire to keep pushing for your dreams. If you or someone close to you has suffered a health crisis, you know how hard it can be to trust in your body again. Worrying about optimal health as you heal can impact your worldview, but you do have a newfound awareness of the possibilities; you've experienced both sides of wellness. Within this expanded context, you can find new levels of happiness in your recovery. Celebrate your body's ability to heal as you focus your energy on a joyful new lease on life.

I feel alive in my body. I thrive in my physical experience and honor the light of possibility in every cell.

REJUVENATION RITUAL

Lie down in the most comfortable space in your home to prepare for bed. Close your eyes and scan your body from your toes to your head, noting any physical tension or pain and transmuting it with rose-gold light and love.

I TRUST MY INNER KNOWING.

Learning how to trust yourself is one of the greatest opportunities available to you, especially after you've been through challenging situations. Do you trust yourself? It's possible you've broken promises with yourself or ignored your intuition (forms of betrayal), affecting your confidence. This week is an opportunity for you to believe in yourself again. Know that your innate wisdom is a guiding light just for you, and it is always available. You can even practice tonight: What does your inner knowing say about the health of your evening routine? Trust your intuition to lead you forward.

My inner knowing is fierce and focused,
aligning with my highest good. This
discernment keeps me from harm—
it is my best guide. I trust myself
fully and wholeheartedly.

REJUVENATION RITUAL

Commune with inner knowing before bed tonight, thinking about a time when you trusted your intuition and you were rewarded. Honor this relationship with love and thanks. (Feels good to have your own back, doesn't it?)

I MAKE CHOICES THAT ALIGN WITH MY LIFE'S VISION.

Every moment is an opportunity to realign with your truth. Are the choices you're making in harmony with your ultimate life vision? If you find yourself feeling trapped between what you want and what is best for those around you, focus on a solution that meets the needs of all involved to the best of your ability. You can still find joy and success in this compromise. When in doubt, ask yourself, *Does this choice make me feel expansive and aligned or heavy and uncomfortable?* Even in your support of others, if you act in alignment with your life's vision, you are ultimately supporting you.

Every choice I make is grounded in love.
I trust myself and my life's vision to live in
integrity and do what is best for all involved.

REJUVENATION RITUAL

In your journal before bed, jot down a big decision that you need to make. Weigh the pros and cons, and as you rest your head on your pillow, focus on the feeling of achieving the outcome you desire.

I RISE ABOVE MY CIRCUMSTANCES; I AM NOT A VICTIM OF THEM.

Many of us bond through our shared experiences. While this is essential to the healing process, if we stay stuck in the pain too long, it becomes part of our identity, taking us further from happiness. There is an opposite phenomenon that can occur after you experience devastation called post-traumatic growth (PTG);[52] instead of becoming the victim of your experience, you emerge the victor. New behaviors, positive thinking, mindset shifts, and reshaping core beliefs are all possible despite hardship. If you are having a difficult time finding solid footing again, start by appreciating the value in your own strength.

I cherish the moments that make me who I am. All of my experiences help me grow into a stronger, wiser person. I am resilient.

REJUVENATION RITUAL

Tonight, write a love letter to yourself. Get creative by using stickers, glitter—whatever you want! Put it in an envelope with a stamp, and give it to a trusted friend this week, asking them to send it to you sometime in the future.

My relationships are healthy and balanced.

Showing up for yourself and showing up for others is grace in action, but helping others when they don't ask for it is doing them a disservice. We all need to learn our own lessons in divine timing. If you are always bailing people out, they learn to rely on you instead of themselves; they don't take accountability. This codependent dynamic weighs on both of you. Tonight, take a look at your relationships to see if they have reciprocal energy. Remember that you don't have to change or fix anything; just allow and accept things as they are, for others as well as yourself. Keep your energy focused on you to attract balanced relationships.

I take care of me, and let others take care of themselves—they do not need to be rescued. I do not engage in relationships at the expense of myself.

REJUVENATION RITUAL

Tonight, revitalize your focus on yourself. Add filtered water and a few drops of peppermint essential oil in a mist bottle, and spray it on your body with love.

I SHARE MY LIFE WITH LOVE AND VULNERABILITY.

Do you shy away from sharing? Being vulnerable is risky, but it can be very rewarding too. When you share more of yourself, you give others permission to share more of themselves, strengthening the bonds between you. Going deeper in outside relationships also deepens the relationship with yourself, because the only way to grow closer to another is to open up more of yourself. If you've ever worried about speaking up out of fear of losing others, you should be more worried about losing yourself. You are the hero of your life's journey, and you have the power to build quality relationships.

I am courageous, sharing my love and vulnerability. I am the hero of my own story, and no one can take this power away from me.

REJUVENATION RITUAL

Commune with yourself through body movement tonight. Put on some music and move your body with the intention of letting go of all judgments and expectations. You can dance, jump on a rebounder, sway, whatever feels good. Embrace the joyful sensations movement gives you.

THE SOUNDS OF NATURE SOOTHE ME.

When is the last time you went outside, gazed at the clouds, and listened to the birds? Did you know that adding this practice to your daily routine could help you sleep better? Listening to the sounds of birds soothes your whole being and supports your nervous system by lowering anxiety, blood pressure, and heart rate.[53] If you have a difficult time falling asleep or you're just looking to relax, consider tuning in to the layered sounds of the natural world. It has the profound capacity to heal us emotionally, mentally, physically, and spiritually, and it's always at the ready—right outside your door.

Nature is my sanctuary, my healer, and my medicine. I listen to its sounds with my entire being. It is my guide to peace—a deep sense of gratitude, calm, and love.

REJUVENATION RITUAL

Listen to bird songs online before bed. Pay attention to how your body feels as its energy shifts, releasing tension and your worries from the day.

I AM NOT THE MISTAKES I'VE MADE.

There's a difference between making mistakes and failing: one embodies growth and the other embodies judgment. Mistakes are labeled "failures" when the ego focuses on the undesired outcome. Consider that there are no mistakes but only learning, and through learning you find growth. After all, you can't make a mistake if you don't have the courage to try, and this is hardly a failure! Listen to your heart, and you'll find that the way things unfolded was the only way to learn the lesson—your personal development opportunity! View your mistakes with compassion to free the wealth of their wisdom.

I have clarity, especially in life's contrasts.
I trust in myself, and my life is as it should be.
There are no mistakes; there's only growth.

REJUVENATION RITUAL

Tonight, start a "fun box" for when you're feeling disillusioned and need a pick-me-up. Put kind words people have said to you in it, photos of loved ones and fun memories, and mementos of your life so far—whatever makes you happy.

Let it begin with my manifestation.

If you feel off track or a little behind in life, it could be that you're comparing yourself to other people—has jealousy hit again? At its core, when you feel jealous of others, it's a reflection of a deep desire that you have yet to meet or else there would be no reaction. Next time jealousy raises its ugly head, rather than allowing resentment to take over, say, "Thank you, Universe, for showing me what is possible." Don't wait for happiness to come to you; start now by aligning yourself to the steps that will take you there. Use this inspiration to manifest your highest path of alignment.

I manifest from a place of alignment.
My inner world is rich with self-discovery,
and I have no need to compare
myself to others.

Rejuvenation Ritual

Realign your energy tonight. Bring one hand to your heart and one to your belly. Sway your body side to side while you invite the energy of self-compassion to fill your body, up from the floor and out the top of your head.

I HAVE THE COURAGE TO TELL THE TRUTH.

People lie for all kinds of reasons—to protect themselves, avoid punishment, impress others—but no matter what, people who lie regularly have low self-esteem; they think telling others what they want to hear will get them what they want. Lying is never a good foundation for a relationship. When we betray the truth, we put ourselves in a psychologically unbalanced state. Self-deception is a sneaky ego trick that keeps you from healing—a false attempt to protect you from pain. Living in delusion may make the moment easier, but it will eventually implode. Find the courage to be honest, especially with yourself. It's the first step to living a life of integrity and authenticity.

I am aligned and in full integrity with myself and others. I am honest because I have self-respect and self-worth.

Rejuvenation Ritual

Put a lapis crystal (associated with honesty, communication, and clarity) under your pillow before bed. As you drift off to sleep, repeat to yourself, *No more lies come from me. All deception from others is blocked from me.*

I RAISE MY VIBRATION IN THE PRESENT TO CREATE A POSITIVE FUTURE.

The rest of your future has yet to be written, though you may spend a lot of time thinking about it. Whether you're fantasizing, daydreaming, or working toward goals, you can miss out on being present with what already *is* when you're too forward focused. Your future is paved by what you do today, and how you show up for yourself each night impacts your tomorrows. Every time you get a good night's sleep, you are investing in your overall well-being, making yourself stronger and healthier for your ideal life. Take clear steps tonight to raise your vibration through a healthier mindset and positive approach to life.

I celebrate my potential by taking care of myself in the moment. I create a solid foundation for a strong future when I raise my vibration in the present.

REJUVENATION RITUAL

Tonight, create a *"my dream life"* positive playlist with songs that motivate you as you work toward manifesting your dreams.

I ALIGN TO MY TRUE INTENTIONS.

Be honest with yourself about the way you've been spending your daily energy. Are there inconsistencies between your intentions and your actions, and if so, what are they? Are you telling yourself one thing but telling other people something else? Do you make promises to yourself but easily flake out as soon as something else comes up? Consider all the ways in which you betray yourself, and consciously focus on healing those aspects—there's a reason you're not following through. As you do this, you will align to your true value, attracting quality connections in your life, especially with yourself. You are worthy of having the life of your dreams.

I honor my true intentions, and I am honest with myself. I listen to my inner voice and trust it to lead me forward. My intentions are pure and trustworthy.

REJUVENATION RITUAL

Have you been getting enough exercise lately? Tonight, make a promise to yourself that you will start exercising regularly and create a plan that starts tomorrow.

I AM AN UNSTOPPABLE FORCE OF CREATIVE WONDER.

Playtime is a fundamental element of childhood, yet as we grow older, we lose sight of its value. We naturally thrive when we are socializing and in a state of flow, but if you're like the 60 percent of American employees who feel like their work–life balance is unhealthy and out of whack,[54] finding time for play is, well, not child's play! Taking the time to do fun things, without an agenda, frees you from the demands of daily life. Research even backs the benefits of doing hobbies, like crafting, gardening—anything that involves creativity, sensory engagement, and self-expression—which are linked to good mental health and well-being.[55] Keep your dopamine and serotonin levels high with more creative projects and playtime.

I love to play and express myself creatively.
I make time for fun and explore the
potential of living in the moment.

REJUVENATION RITUAL

This evening, take out a sketch pad and your markers, crayons, colored pencils, stickers, scrapbook material, etc., and create a fun, mixed-media self-portrait!

I AM A POWERFUL CREATOR OF POSITIVE EXPERIENCES.

Feeling down and out? Well, maybe you can turn that frown completely around! There are many tricks to help you find your happy. You know the value of exercising, getting more sleep, eating a healthy diet, focusing on gratitude, and thinking positively. Unless you're an eternal optimist, however, thinking positive thoughts isn't always realistic. Plus, your brain doesn't know the difference between that fantasy of you finally winning the lottery versus the stark contrast of you wondering how you're going to pay next month's rent. There is a huge gap between what *is* and what *could be*—cognitive dissonance is real. When you focus on positive thinking, always pair it with inspired action, and you'll reach your heart's desires much sooner.

I am happy when I make a habit of positive thinking and focus on what I can control. I am thankful for all my experiences, and I dive into them fully.

REJUVENATION RITUAL

Before bed, jot down in your journal your day's awesome moments, no matter how small.

I AM THE CHAMPION OF MY DEEPEST DESIRES AND DREAMS.

Are you working toward a goal but doubting its possibility? Did you create the vision board and talk about your dream, but still, the reality isn't here? If you're feeling stuck, try applying the universal law of inspired action, where you take real, actionable steps to invite what you want into your life. Daily action reaps the reward. But here are the most important steps: intentionally slow down, get quiet, and create space for internal guidance to support your process. When we let go of our need to control the outcome, we open to it and even more possibilities, achieving our goals and beyond.

I focus on moving closer to what I desire by slowing down and getting quiet. I take inspired action when it feels right to do so. I live in the energy of my heart's desires.

REJUVENATION RITUAL

Align with your heart's desires before bed. Light a stick of incense, close your eyes, tune in to your breathing, and intuitively feel in to your next inspired action.

I CREATE MY REALITY.

People become uncomfortable for two reasons in life: (1) they are staying in their comfort zone but have outgrown it, or (2) they have left their comfort zone and everything around them is new and unfamiliar. No matter where you are in your life's journey, you get to create the reality you desire. Instead of making choices from a place of outside demands, choose to align to your soul's desires. What lights it up? What are you passionate about? Make choices that feel inspiring to you. You create more magnificent opportunities by identifying what you want clearly and then embodying that energy *right now.*

My life is a beautiful manifestation of my truest intentions and desires. The lifestyle I embody is in accordance with my vision for a life well lived.

REJUVENATION RITUAL

Tonight, treat yourself to something sweet as you practice intentional action. Focus on the experience before you even begin eating, taking in the scent, shape, and taste memory. Get clear on what you're calling in, then relax your mind and enjoy.

I AM COMMITTED TO FULFILLING MY LIFE'S PURPOSE.

You're on a rapid healing journey on a highway of awesomeness, charging away from your past and into your bright future—make sure you wear your shades! When you move forward, away from what you've known, you may start to ponder your purpose and if you are living your life the "right" way. Your purpose is not something you need to find or chase—it lives inside of you already. You have a unique set of skills, talents, and ideas that are yours alone; when you use and honor them, you activate them—you live with purpose. Living with purpose *is* your life's purpose. Fill each day with this purpose, and you'll never go astray.

I honor all aspects of myself—I feel abundant and purposeful. With each intentional choice, I am more at ease.

REJUVENATION RITUAL

Tonight, make up your own rhythmic chanting while you do something you love. Align your voice to your enjoyment of the activity, and experience the expansive resonance it creates.

I RESPECT AND PROTECT MYSELF.

No one has the power to make you feel a specific way except for you, so if you feel like you are trying to prove yourself to others, change your focus from the insecurity of lack to the security of abundance. Fill yourself with more love instead. When you're strong within—when you respect yourself and know your worth—what others do and say does not affect you, and you no longer question yourself. Moving forward, surround yourself with people who see your value and respect you as you are. Just remember that *you* set the example—it starts with you seeing and protecting your own worth.

I see myself through the lens of love. I take care of and protect myself at all costs. I have nothing to prove—I am enough. I give myself the respect I want from others.

REJUVENATION RITUAL

Before bed, reflect in your journal on the ways you respect and protect yourself. What are your favorite qualities?

I THRIVE UNDER PRESSURE, SHINING BRIGHT LIKE A DIAMOND.

No one wants a life of challenges, but the truth is, life is full of them. Fortunately, they come with a choice: to see difficulties as opportunities for learning and growth or to succumb to the pressure. Doing hard things requires resiliency and inner strength to show us what we're made of.

You can only become a diamond through experiencing condensed pressure in your life. This pressure builds character, transforming your being into the brightest version of you. When life's challenges are intense and the pressure's mounting, apply more love to make things easier. The challenges may still be present, but the love releases the valve so you prevail.

Life's pressures take me to higher ground— to greater clarity and strength. I thrive in new situations and shine bright like the diamond I am.

REJUVENATION RITUAL

Sit comfortably in a space where the moonlight is visible tonight (or visualize its bright light). Close your eyes and feel the moon's diamond rays rejuvenating your body, mind, and spirit.

332

My abundance and wealth are always increasing.

When you earn money, how does it feel? In contrast, how does it feel when you pay your bills? Money flows where intention goes, with a consciousness and vibrational frequency to it. It doesn't matter if the money's coming or going; your internal experience of it impacts your wealth trajectory. How you think about, spend, and save money are all part of your abundance mindset. This includes the money mindset and subconscious beliefs of your caretakers that were passed on to you through their own behaviors and conditioned patterns. If a scarcity mindset is limiting your manifestation abilities, it's time to balance your abundance mentality with self-worth and self-love.

Abundance is the language of my heart.
When I align to the vibration of love,
its wealth multiplies tenfold.

Rejuvenation Ritual

Before bed, place any spare bills and coins on the windowsill. Fall asleep thinking about how you will spend the money with gratitude, trusting that it will return to you tenfold.

I AM OPEN TO RECEIVING ALL THE GOOD AROUND ME.

When you feel depleted, it's difficult to find motivation. If you're not allowing yourself to be in receiving energy, you will feel even more exhausted from overexerting yourself. There's a yin and yang to all opportunities and situations. When you give, allow yourself to also receive, and when you receive, be open to giving. See the support that comes your way as little gifts from the universe and giving back as returning the favor. There's a balance to the ebbs and flows of your life. Tonight, retract your energy and allow yourself to receive the goodness that is always available to you.

When I sleep, I receive good energy. I am open to receiving more love and support to balance the love and support I give.

REJUVENATION RITUAL

Connect with Earth's abundant energy tonight by stepping outside with bare feet and touching the ground, even if it's for a short while. You can also enhance your abundance vibes by investing in a Chinese money tree or bamboo plant for your home.

I AM THE BEST VERSION OF MYSELF TODAY.

If you feel off track, take the bird's-eye view on any situation that is causing you stress. Use this vantage point to see the opportunities you have to change course in a direction that feels more aligned. Redirect yourself to protect yourself. How do you want to live your life? How do you talk to yourself about this? When you focus on living life in exciting ways, life can be passionate again. Just remember to be kind to yourself—you're doing the best you can. Be open to new experiences, focus on what you want to create, and be an enthusiastic cheerleader along the way. Embrace your best self every day.

My life is beautiful because of the loving choices I make. I expand myself to receive opportunities that were previously unknown and unimaginable. My best self is my daily self.

REJUVENATION RITUAL

Before bed tonight, step away from your daily perspective to take a different view. Write down the ways you could make improvements and what you want to manifest this week.

MY CONFIDENCE GROWS FROM CHALLENGING EXPERIENCES.

Healing is not linear, and there is no official destination. When you are going through darkness, all you can do is look for the light. Recognize that you are in the shadows of life—it's not permanent. Like the dark of each night, these shadows eventually fade and light returns. When trauma occurs, your sense of safety is threatened, clouding your lens of the world and your ability to trust others. But this is your path to wholeness. Confidence comes from surviving these experiences and the depths of understanding that come from them. You learn that you matter—you didn't let trauma dictate your worth! You made it through and deserve to stand tall.

I am here for a reason, and I am valuable.
As I grow and heal, my confidence expands.
My power is my purpose.

REJUVENATION RITUAL

Is your bedroom your haven? Assess your sleep space tonight, and if you haven't already, turn it into your sanctuary with whatever is positive and peaceful to you (candles, inspirational quotes, photographs of loved ones, etc.).

I MAKE SMALL SHIFTS FOR BIG RESULTS.

People are creatures of habit, and we fall into routines that feel safe, comfortable, and satisfactory. Find safety in your bedtime routine too. Preparing yourself for bed activates your brain to begin winding down for rest mode. As you set yourself up for a good night's sleep, your brain recognizes that you are safe and your body can relax. Look at your current prebedtime habits: Where is there an opportunity for improvement? Make small shifts to reap larger, lasting results. Be intentional with your bedtime routine to improve your sleep health overall, one step and one night at a time.

I experiment with my evening routine to maximize its benefits. I focus on small changes that are manageable and enjoyable, so I can rest more peacefully and well.

REJUVENATION RITUAL

At bedtime, crawl into bed and wiggle your toes. This is one small thing that triggers relaxation as you actively release tension from the day.

My time is incredibly valuable–I know my worth.

If you are transitioning from one life phase into another, perhaps reentering the dating pool or embarking on a new career path, make sure to tune your intention to your heart. If your self-worth is directed elsewhere, you might take an easy job that doesn't challenge you or choose a partner who's good on paper but not in action. When self-worth is tied to the outside world, we make choices that keep us small, because we feel bad about ourselves. Make a promise to yourself that moving forward, you'll value yourself by aiming higher, going after goals that are worthy of *you* and nothing less.

My time and energy are important.
I show my worth through the choices I make
and opportunities I accept—I settle
for nothing less.

Rejuvenation Ritual

At bedtime, put a few drops of jasmine perfume or essential oil on your wrists and your heart chakra. Breathe in the fragrance deeply while focusing on feeling beautiful, whole, and priceless—the greatest treasures in your life.

I PUT MYSELF FIRST, TO ALIGN WITH LOVE AND CARE.

Do you give love with a desperate undertone? Do you try to earn love or give away your power to choose? When efforts in love are not reciprocated, some instinctively try harder instead of smarter. This cycle depletes your energy and builds up resentment. For example, if you overwork to gain your partner's approval but they don't value your efforts, they are taking advantage, exploiting your time or energy. No amount of energy, love, and time dedicated to those who lack appreciation will equal the same outcome in return. Put yourself first, never giving more than what you are receiving.

I put my needs first to align with love and care. How I show up for me is how I best show up for others and receive the same love in return.

REJUVENATION RITUAL

Practice belly breathing before bed. Place your hands on your diaphragm and feel it expand and contract as you breathe deeply. Focus on the energy of love moving through your body, throughout your entire home, and back again.

I TRUST DIVINE TIMING– ALL IS IN PERFECT ORDER.

Have you been focusing on what you currently don't have instead of what you do? This comes from a place of ego insecurity that says there is not enough in the world to meet your needs, giving this fear more power. If it feels like what you need is not here, ask yourself honestly, *Is this a need or a want?* We always get what we need in life, but it may not look like what we want. When you recognize how good things are already, you imbue more clarity in your manifestations. Focus on what you want and be thankful for having all that you need.

I honor my needs by honoring what is going well. All is in perfect order, and I am grateful.

REJUVENATION RITUAL

Tonight, light some sage or copal and walk around your house to cleanse the space. Open a window or door with the intention that the smoke ushers your burdens outside, to the night sky. (Make sure the sage or copal is extinguished before bed.)

I WELCOME UNEXPECTED ABUNDANCE.

When you start a new workout routine, it may take time to see results, but in time, if you don't give up, you'll pass that threshold and see all your hard work paying off. When it comes to working with your higher self, however, having faith in the unexpected is important. You must trust your higher power and the energy of the universe, believing in the magic of unexpected opportunities. Focus on the frequency of abundance and bask in this energy. As you do, you show the universe that you are available to receive in fun and creative ways.

I support myself by supporting my visions.
I open myself to the universe and its
magic to manifest abundance beyond my
wildest dreams.

REJUVENATION RITUAL

Tonight, consider how you can focus on prosperity through the choices you make this week. For example, switch out your regular water bottle for one of colored glass, or buy yourself a bouquet of flowers. Get creative by gifting yourself with a few surprises too.

I EMBODY PEACE.

Everybody on the planet has access to divinity; true peace and fulfillment do not come from anything outside of yourself. If you're dependent on outside influences to feel good, this is an illusion of your fear-based mind. Realize that your greatest happiness fix is not in the next job, the next paycheck, the next relationship, the next like on social media; true happiness and fulfillment come from within your true self. One way to boost your happiness is to step away from your online habits tonight. Know that the power of peaceful presence lies within, and honor it daily. It is your ever-present source of divinity, balance, abundance, and peace.

Peace is my purpose and my energy, and I align to it every night. My choices embody peace as I embody peace.

REJUVENATION RITUAL

Plan a social-media detox this week. Could you reduce your habits to just checking in once a day and turn off the notifications on your phone? Make it realistic for you and then see how it makes you feel.

ABUNDANT BLESSINGS COME TO ME WITH EASE.

Tonight, as you prepare for bed, you have an opportunity to practice nonjudgment. Accept what is—*all* of it. Neutralize your emotional attachment to anything that vibrationally brings you down. Focus on retracting your energy from situations that you feel you have no control or power over. From this place, you live in a neutral state, with much more powerful attracting energy. There is no resistance, and what you want comes easily to you. Accept what is and embrace all your abundant blessings now, and those that have yet to come.

I manifest from a place of love and abundance, for all that I desire is already here within me. I trust the process and embrace everything as it is.

REJUVENATION RITUAL

As you turn down your bed tonight, turn inward to think about your blessings—big and small, obvious and overlooked. List five in your journal that resonate the most, then fall asleep with gratitude to the universe.

343

I VALUE MY FANTASIES AND ALIGN THEM TO TRUTH.

Sometimes we want something, but we don't take action toward it because we fall into the notion of *if it's meant for me, it won't pass me by.* But the truth is that in order to get what you want, you need to put forth consistent effort. Expecting your fantasies to fall into your lap without effort on your part leans toward hubris energy. Hubris is excessive confidence, extreme pride, and arrogance. If you feel entitled to what you want and expect it to be yours without any work, you are only hurting yourself. Instead, go inward, connect with your ancestors, and ask, *What is the next inspired action I can take that is for my highest good?* Let your vision lead you to a life you desire with grounded action and guidance from your lineage.

I take guided action and align my desires with the guidance of my ancestors. I am in control of my life and take action toward my desires.

REJUVENATION RITUAL

In your journal, identify a dream or goal you want to manifest and list out any ego barriers (assumptions or fears) you suspect may get in the way. Now list out a few inspired action steps you can take this week toward your desire.

WE ARE ALL MADE OF THE STARS. WE ARE ONE.

The most fundamental law of the universe is the Law of Divine Oneness, which honors the interconnectedness of all things. It's the idea that beyond our senses, every thought, action, and event is connected to everything else—like the six degrees of separation theory times infinity. If everything is connected and we all come from the same place, consider all that exists to be like family. Approach all situations with the question, *How can I show more compassion and acceptance toward those I don't understand?* or *What would divine love do?* From this level of connection, you'll dwell in peace and harmony.

I am one with all that exists, connected by the love and the stardust we are made of. I extend compassion to all my brothers and sisters, on Earth and beyond.

REJUVENATION RITUAL

Say a prayer for the planet before bed: "May all the beings on Earth flourish in the love that they are. Help them to find their light and realize their highest potential. *Namaste.*"

I RISE WITH LOVE AND JOY.

Do you fall asleep in a positive mental space and rise in one too, or do you feel stressed when you lay your head down to sleep and wake up still feeling anxious? How you rise in the morning is directly related to how you fall asleep. Taking time to perform bedtime routines grounded in love and self-compassion will help you wake up with more appreciation and wonder, making you feel better overall. Choose to rise in love by celebrating the joyful things around you right now, especially the simple little things that easily get passed by. Take time tonight to set yourself up for a better day tomorrow.

I make conscious choices each night
to positively impact my day tomorrow.
Gratitude, joy, and love are my
bedtime focus.

REJUVENATION RITUAL

Before bed, make a list of five everyday things that you're grateful for—things that are easily taken for granted. Leave this list nearby, so that it's one of the first things you see in the morning.

REST IS AN OPPORTUNITY TO IMAGINE, DISCOVER, AND CREATE.

Do you need a little physical breather, or do you just want a mini mental escape? Our minds need a vacation too. Do you give yourself permission to daydream? Not only can it inspire new perspectives, but daydreaming feels better than forcing yourself to find a solution when you feel stuck in solving a problem. Research proves that mind-wandering can boost the cognitive process, inspiring new perspectives and creativity.[56] Daydreaming taps into your childlike sense of wonder, an energy of innocence and curiosity takes over, and you have more fun with the possibilities. This imaginative view of life will help you feel more at ease as you allow your creative juices to flow. Take this with you to bed tonight to inspire yourself to dream.

I tap into my ideas and inspiration tonight.
I rest peacefully knowing that my creative self
is nurtured and cared for.

REJUVENATION RITUAL

Tonight, get creative in the kitchen with a recipe from a beloved cookbook or from online by adding your own signature touch.

I AM A STAR AND MY OWN GUIDING LIGHT.

It's smart to have a ten-year plan and a daily to-do list, but being too serious about life has its drawbacks. If you think back to some of the most rewarding times so far, the spontaneous moments may be the ones that have really stayed in your heart. Finding a healthy balance between routine and wonder is a skill we can cultivate daily. The key to living a fulfilling life is to focus on what you want, putting loving intention toward it, and then enjoying the freedom for it to come to you. Shine your own light forward, letting your heart illuminate the way.

I am unapologetic about my inner light and radiate with love for myself. I take care of the star that I am and trust in its guidance.

REJUVENATION RITUAL

As you lie in bed tonight, visualize a large, cobalt-blue orb of energy in front of you. Imagine stepping forward into the bubble so that you are fully inside of it. Drift off to sleep knowing you are radiant and protected.

I DETACH FROM THE DAILY HUSTLE AND FIND SOLACE IN MYSELF.

The daily hustle culture has an undertone of need—need for validation, appreciation, attention, admiration—and it's weak with false illusions, a tower that will eventually crumble. Burnout, disease, mental-health issues, relationship toxicity, and sleep disorders are just some of the threats at every turn. If your life is built on validation through the path of working harder, there is no end in sight. Even if you love what you do and are passionate about your career, honoring your basic needs is critical: quality sleep, healthy food, movement and exercise, love and connection. Make sure you give yourself time to rest and enjoy some solace, free of work's demands.

Decompressing each night is as important as breathing. I practice mindfulness and seek to live my life in a harmonious, self-nurturing way.

REJUVENATION RITUAL

Before bed, connect with your presence in the moment. Close your eyes, breathe into your body, and ask yourself, *Where do I seek validation outside of myself? How can I give myself that which I seek?* And start to do this tomorrow.

I AM THE SUPERHERO IN MY LIFE STORY.

There's an infamous allure to superheroes—these pop-culture characters are popular for good reason! Brave and self-sacrificing, they use their abilities to ward off evil forces and protect the innocent. Who wouldn't love these aspirational leaders? The problem with superheroes is that most of them wear a disguise to conceal their identity—to protect themselves from the world and its sinister forces. If they can't be their full, true selves (which always causes internal conflict, by the way), can they be real superheroes? Recognize that your own full self is enough—the most powerful force there is! If you are struggling within, consider showing more of your true self in your life. Don't compartmentalize; just be you and shine.

I take off my mask to be my true self in all areas of my life. It is my greatest power against difficulty, and my resilience is my mentor.

REJUVENATION RITUAL

Tonight, plan out a week's worth of outfits that make you feel confident and unstoppable—you are a powerful, mighty force!

I AM A LIVING MIRACLE.

You are a miracle! As you move forward in your life, embrace this realization with every part of your being. It can be a tough feat to look for the good and miraculous when you're feeling down and defeated, but you can train yourself to do this much, like training any muscle in the body. Recognizing a miracle requires a shift in perception, so look at this practice as an opportunity to celebrate the good, no matter what! See yourself and others in all your gorgeous glory. The fact that you are breathing right now is a blessing in itself. Fall asleep embracing the miracle that you are.

I am light and I am love. I see the miracle of each moment and embody this. Self-love is my gift to the universe and others.

REJUVENATION RITUAL

Tonight, take a hot bubble bath and feel the warm flow of the water. Celebrate the miracle of your life and your soul— you are a one-of-a-kind product of divinity!

I MAKE SPACE FOR LOVE, ABUNDANCE, AND PROSPERITY.

If you have a parent, friend, or romantic partner who has violated your trust, you've felt the trauma of betrayal. This type of insidious pain impacts self-esteem, other relationships, and your emotional health. If you're going through a heartbreak, put your trust in your healing—it *will* get easier with time. The best thing you can do now is to take care of you, creating space for love. Prioritizing self-care means being your own best friend and cherishing your beautiful self. As you take care of you, in time, your heart will open again. Believe in yourself and trust in love—the path to abundance and prosperity.

Every experience helps me grow into my destiny. Abundance and love flow effortlessly to me. I am free to receive prosperity.

REJUVENATION RITUAL

Spend time tonight doing *il dolce far niente*, which is Italian for "the sweetness of doing nothing." It's the art of seeking pleasure in the pause of every idle moment. Embrace it fully.

I REST SAFELY IN MY BODY, TRUSTING ALL IS WELL.

Next time you feel triggered, take a moment to check in before reacting—where do you feel this reaction coming up in you? Your body will often have a response physically, emotionally, or both. Pay attention to the triggers too—why does your body feel unsafe? When we recognize that our mind is replaying a projection from the past into the present, we can pause the overreaction to the trigger. To protect your peace, start to nurture your body to build a stronger relationship with it. Your body is a master at protecting you, so pay attention to its valuable clues.

I trust myself to recognize and understand my triggers. I am safe and well in my body.

REJUVENATION RITUAL

Before bed, visualize something that makes you feel safe and comfortable (love from another person, a special blanket, calming music, etc.), and mentally wrap yourself in it. Remember that you can access this safety anytime you feel triggered; you are your own master protector.

I TAKE ACTION TO CREATE PEACE IN THE WORLD.

Altruistic behavior is virtuous, but not all of us abide by it. Some people see the act of giving as only a means of receiving, so their interactions are transactional—they're thinking about what's in it for them. But pure altruism is found by taking compassionate action without expecting anything in return. It's also a way to boost your happy brain chemicals, which are associated with the pleasure and reward centers in your brain. So the next time you feel hopeless about the state of suffering in the world, you can immediately relieve that despair by helping others in need.

I invite more love into the world through intentional acts of love and care. I support those in need with my time, resources, energy, and love without expectation. I create the peace I desire in the world.

REJUVENATION RITUAL

Flex your altruism muscles tonight by researching how you can support a local homeless shelter, food pantry, children's hospital, or animal shelter—whatever cause resonates with you.

I EXPLORE MY INNER WORLD OF UNTAPPED POTENTIAL.

Spend time exploring your unconscious behaviors and habits, such as self-defeating thoughts, unprocessed anger, and compulsive patterns of quick gratification. The behaviors outside of your conscious awareness can negatively impact your ability to have a healthy, fulfilling life. What's getting in the way of your untapped potential? Do you have attitudes that cloud your perspective and compassion? Do you believe you're worthy of your dreams? Anything that is too painful to process gets stuffed into your unconscious mind and affects your entire being. Identify the roots of your distress by getting curious. Use techniques like dream analysis and free association to start healing and unblock the divine flow of your potential.

I go deeper into my unconscious to access healing and strength. I bravely explore my inner world of untapped potential to unlock the power of my dreams.

REJUVENATION RITUAL

Lying in bed tonight, tap your third eye with your pointer finger as you visualize opening a direct communication channel with your subconscious mind. Ask yourself what blocks are hindering your potential.

355

I JOYFULLY SHOW THE WORLD WHO I AM.

Many of us hide behind false personalities to protect ourselves, such as the overachiever who craves praise, the self-defeated person who puts themselves down before others can, the avoidant one who rejects others before they get rejected, the conformer who craves belonging, and the people pleaser who desperately serves others for acceptance. We all have needs that we aim to fulfill through our personalities, but this is not the source of authenticity. Being authentic is being aligned with your core values, being self-aware, and honoring and embodying your beliefs and psychological needs. Make sure you are showing up as your true self by aligning *who* you are with *how* you are in the world.

Everything within me honors my values and my truth. I live in alignment with my heart and my soul—authenticity is my great joy.

REJUVENATION RITUAL

Tonight, light a candle with loving intention. Write five "I am" statements in your journal in honor of the true you.

TRANQUILITY IS MY REFUGE.

Every thought that you have has an energetic vibration tied to it. When you focus on love, you create a ripple effect in the universe—putting out positivity attracts good things back to you. You have a powerful opportunity to feel healed and whole, and it comes rooted in the energy of love. By keeping your vibration high, you have more composure and peace. Tonight, focus on love's healing vibration to bring tranquil balance to your life. When you radiate love with your intentions and thoughts, you contribute to the collective energy of abundance and joy. Crown yourself with divine love.

Every thought I have sends out a magnetic
resonance and vibration to the world,
uplifting all with more joy and peace,
including myself. I focus my thoughts on
healing and hope.

REJUVENATION RITUAL

Before bed, sit in a chair with your feet directly under your knees at a ninety-degree angle, with a neutral spine. Visualize and energetically feel the crown of your head lifting upward toward the heavens, connecting to the universal energy of divine love. Imagine an actual crown on your head and relax deeper into your sovereign divine royalty.

I AM THE GATEKEEPER TO MY EMOTIONS AND THEIR ENERGIES.

The next time a person pops into your mind, consider sending them a prayer of goodwill. If they continually come to mind, they might just be thinking of you too. If negative feelings come up when you think about someone, recognize where this lives in your body. Is it from a bad experience in your past? Don't dwell on it; instead, acknowledge the emotional expression and release it. When you ruminate, you bypass the healing presenting itself. Feel the emotions in your body and act as their gatekeeper, releasing those that bring your energy down, attuning to the ones that feel uplifting, and thanking all experiences for their lessons.

I am the gatekeeper to my emotional landscape. I release what doesn't serve me and heal myself with love.

REJUVENATION RITUAL

Tonight, go outside—into your yard or on your deck—or look out your window at a star or simply envision one. Identify a negative thought that you've had recently and send it to the star. Watch it transmute the pain into peace and release it to the heavens.

Healing requires taking responsibility.

We model the behavior we see growing up. If you grew up with emotionally unavailable caretakers, you may find yourself in emotionally unavailable partnerships. When you wake up to a higher level of awareness, you start to see that your internal lens has been rooted in insecure wounds. As you heal, you no longer accept what you once settled for; you see your worth and feel more empowered as you take responsibility for your life circumstances. You see that everyone is on their own healing journey, and others who act from a wounded place are still unaware of it. Your vision is clear, and you love them with all your healed heart.

I work with intention to heal the wounded parts of me. I am committed to being strong, healthy, and happy.

Rejuvenation Ritual

Before bed, write in your journal about a situation in which you hurt someone else, even if it was unintentional. What is the unhealed wound within that is reflected by this experience? Explore that as you send this person a prayer of love.

I CONSCIOUSLY CALM THE CHAOS IN MY MIND.

When you seek answers in life, do you have the quiet mental space for receiving the guidance that comes? If you are stuck in a statie mental loop, this chaotic prison can lead to mental health issues, performance and relationship problems, and sleep disturbances. People with mental health and sleep disorders say intrusive thoughts make it tougher to get good shut-eye, even more so than experiences of physical pain.[57] If you struggle to sleep, distracting yourself with imaginary scenarios can help. For example, if you're worried about an upcoming work presentation, imagine yourself not only nailing it but getting the high fives from your entire team afterward. Immerse yourself in feel-good scenarios and drift off to sleep with less effort.

Mental rest is my focus and peace. A calm mind is an open mind—a place where intuition thrives.

REJUVENATION RITUAL

Tonight, go on a much-needed vacation in your mind. Immerse yourself in the sounds, textures, smells, and sights of this place, imagining it as deeply as you can until you feel at peace.

I DON'T HAVE TO BE PERFECT TO BE LOVED.

Have you been getting down on yourself, saying *I don't deserve to be happy, or I feel like an imposter*? You're not alone. Studies show more than 70 percent of people secretly worry they are not good enough.[58] What looks like perfectionism could be a desperate fear of failure and vulnerability at its root. If you're a perfectionist, you are likely terrified of making mistakes, overworking to cover up your shortcomings. But this is a vicious cycle where fear feeds false belief, making you more exhausted and afraid than ever. Wave the white flag and see that your perceived "flaws" are actually what make you lovable. You are human, and your humanity—the humble, raw part of you—is your strength.

I let go of my need to control and accept what is. The current moment is perfect, and I am lovable exactly as I am.

REJUVENATION RITUAL

Silence your inner meanie by creating a feel-good file before bed, filling it with photos, cartoons, notes from loved ones— whatever makes you feel good about yourself.

I FORGIVE, AND I AM FORGIVEN.

When you've been wronged by another person, can you see them as your teacher? Detach from the experience to see its exchange of energy. Pay attention to how you relate to the person—is it an energy of betrayal, guilt, shame? Feelings are energy, and some studies theorize that consciousness is comprised of organized energy in the brain.[59] Work on forgiving yourself and others by understanding the lessons of this energy—something in your auric field attracted the other person's consciousness to help you learn, heal, and grow. For example, if you have a fear of rejection and get ghosted, this is an opportunity to heal wounded energy. The opposite of forgiveness is stagnation; forgive to move forward and grow.

I forgive myself for the pain I cause others,
and I forgive others to release resentment.
Forgiveness allows me to move forward
and grow.

REJUVENATION RITUAL

Tonight, light two candles to represent you and a person you wish to forgive. Repeat the Hawaiian Ho'oponopono prayer: "I'm sorry—please forgive me. Thank you. I love you."[60]

I AM WORTH THE LIFE I DESIRE.

What is the dream in your heart that has yet to be actualized? Whatever the desire, it most likely keeps coming back, over and over—it is a dream that is meant to be realized through you in this lifetime. You are worth your ideal life, and the problems that keep interfering are just obstacles to overcome and make you stronger. See any blockages as opportunities to release what doesn't fit into the vision of the dream you're working toward. It's time to take hold of the vision you have for your life and manifest it. You are worth the life of your dreams.

Any problems, burdens, or situations that come between my dreams and me are released with intention. I show up with passion and love to manifest my dream.

REJUVENATION RITUAL

Before bed, close your eyes and identify an obstacle in your life. Picture rose-gold light pouring into the situation and flooding it with love. As you release the problem to higher realms, you remove the barrier for good.

I COMMIT TO MY DESIRED PATH AND FOCUS ON MY PURPOSE.

When you focus on your intentions and lead from your value system, you manifest a reality that supports your overall well-being. In contrast, when you make choices out of fear, you often do so without realizing the consequences, causing regret, frustration, and overwhelm. To reclaim your personal power and feel more aligned to your true self, focus on the visions you have for your life. Continually check in with yourself—what kind of life do you really want to live? Align each choice to your bigger vision, and every choice will be easier to make. You are either contributing to your vision or deterring from it. Honor your dreams by being intentional with each choice you make.

I create my ideal life by aligning with my bigger vision. Every choice brings me closer to my dreams.

REJUVENATION RITUAL

Identify a dream that you are working toward. What decision can you make tonight to move closer toward manifesting this desire? Write it down so you don't forget!

REWARDING DREAMS AWAIT ME.

Something within you knows you were made for more. Living a life of purpose and passion comes down to fulfillment, and living a fulfilled life means you're following through on your dreams—you're taking actions to manifest the desires in your heart. Don't worry about how it will look to other people or if it will even work out; just commit yourself to the dream. Take steps toward it and believe in it, and soon, your dream will manifest into reality. As you live a life of fulfillment, you start to realize the depths of your growth and potential. The dreams you have are awaiting you, and it is your mission and opportunity to go for them.

I go for my dreams and honor them by taking daily steps toward their fulfillment. My heart overflows with love when I follow through on its desires.

REJUVENATION RITUAL

Reorient your evening routine to include a creative planning session with dice or a flip of a coin. Freshen up tomorrow's to-do list by rolling the dice, or using a coin, to determine the order of your tasks, or make sure to add fun breaks in between.

CHANGING MY MIND AS NEEDED MAKES ME STRONG, NOT WEAK.

If you struggle to make decisions and feel pressure to optimize every choice, you could be stuck in a cycle of decision fatigue. To get a better perspective, distance yourself from the problem. Working on other projects, going for a walk—anything you can do to change directions will stop the cycle of fixation and lead you toward resolution. Give yourself the space to go inward and listen to your intuition. You can change your mind at any time without judgment. Make choices based on what feels best for you versus what you think is right or wrong.

I am confident in my choices—they serve my highest good. I am strong when I focus on what is best for me and follow through.

REJUVENATION RITUAL

Test your intuition tonight by flipping a coin. Allocate each side to an option for a choice you need to make, then see if it lands on heads or tails. Pay attention to how you feel with the result, and what your intuitive nudge felt like before the result, then choose the option that feels best.

I QUESTION MY ASSUMPTIONS WITH SINCERITY.

No matter how wonderful a relationship seems, there are always conflicts and areas of communication that can be addressed. Sometimes we put invisible demands on our loved ones without even realizing it. You loan your friend money with the expectation that they'll pay you back, or you do extra chores with the expectation you will get more affection in return. These unspoken agreements rooted in assumptions are called covert contracts, and they are invisible relationship saboteurs, leading to misunderstandings and resentment, to name a few. To maintain healthier relationships, start by looking at expectations of your own that have not been directly expressed. Be sincere with yourself, and you will see a positive shift in your relationship dynamics.

I am honest with myself and transparent with others. I communicate my needs and expectations clearly and encourage others to do the same.

REJUVENATION RITUAL

Get honest with yourself tonight about some unspoken expectations you have with a loved one. Make steps toward alleviating the imbalance this week by first apologizing, then sharing your plan to remedy it.

I PRACTICE SELF-LOVE BY HONORING MY BOUNDARIES.

When you focus on inner peace, things start to shift in your world. You no longer pay attention to outside dramas or conflict, and you cut out the people who are stuck, focusing on your own growth instead. Set the bar high for yourself and invite those around you to do the same; if they decline, wish them well and be on your way. Once on a personal path of growth, you feel stronger, healthier, and wiser—keep your evolution going! Implement a boundary for anyone taking your energy; yours is a path of peace and purpose. Nothing can take you off your path.

I honor the flow of my life and go where I feel supported and loved. I am committed to growth and peace, and I invite others to join me. I release all attachment.

REJUVENATION RITUAL

Before bed, grab some prayer beads or a prayer stone and hold it in your hands. Identify a relationship you are ready to release, give it love, then hand it over to the universe or your higher power.

REGARDLESS OF THE OUTCOME, I AM TAKEN CARE OF BY LOVE.

Everyone knows someone whose behaviors are incredibly rude or disrespectful, yet they blame others for their actions. People who don't take accountability wreak havoc in life. Protect your peace of mind by not enabling this behavior. When you separate yourself from these dynamics, you feel more grounded and clear. Wanting justice is motivating, but letting karma do her thing is best—it's the inescapable spiritual law that balances all of life. Whatever we put out into the universe comes back to us—*always*. As you sow, so shall you reap.

I am always taken care of by the universe in love when I demonstrate, embody, and give love. I focus on what I can control and let karma take care of the rest.

REJUVENATION RITUAL

Put the powers of love to work tonight by sending blessings or prayers to a challenging person in your life. Conclude the practice by lighting some sage and giving the rest to the universe's care.

SOME OF MY GREATEST MEMORIES ARE STILL TO COME.

When you free your mind of past worries and future fears, all that's left is the present moment, where your personal power is amplified. Your creative potential and your divine flow state live in this moment—this is the access point to your true self. Focus on your dreams to create a life in alignment with your values. It takes optimism and courage, but you have both flooding through your veins. Look forward to the life yet to be lived by planting the seeds of tomorrow *today*.

If it doesn't serve me, I cut ties with it.
I focus on what I want and know it wants me
too. I love my life as it is and look forward
to the moments yet to come.

REJUVENATION RITUAL

Before bed, meditate on something that you've always wanted to do but haven't given yourself permission to pursue. Visualize yourself moving forward on this dream, and make a tangible plan to manifest it into reality.

I AWAKEN FROM MY DREAM STATE AND ASCEND INTO UNCONDITIONAL LOVE.

When you are clear within your own self about who you are and what you want in your life, you have awakened from your dream state. No longer sleepwalking, you realize that our world pushes concepts, beliefs, and ideals that are the opposite of your true divine nature. Instead of allowing the outside world to force its agenda on you, reclaim your personal autonomy by accessing the wisdom of your heart and taking responsibility for your life. This is where freedom resides. Live the life you never could have imagined for yourself prior to your awakening.

I am free of limiting programming and beliefs. I awaken from my sleep state to ascend into the realm of my highest potential.

REJUVENATION RITUAL

Tonight, light a candle in honor of your true self, giving yourself gratitude for being who you are and for the things you love about yourself. When you blow out the candle before going to sleep, release these loving thoughts to softly mingle with your dreams.

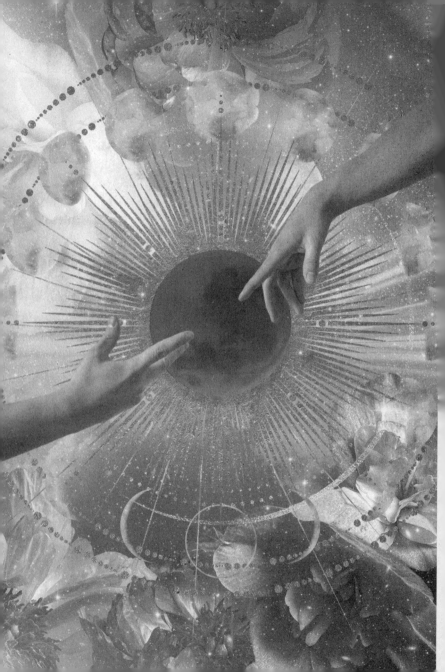

ACKNOWLEDGMENTS

The process of bringing this book to life was an incredible journey, and I am forever grateful for the transformation it has brought about. Thank you, Michele Ashtiani Cohn and Richard Cohn at Beyond Words for bringing this book idea to me and presenting it to Simon & Schuster. Thank you to my fantastic book agent, Steve Harris, for the option to design and bring the partner deck *Happy Bedtime Mantras Card Deck* into the world. I appreciate my editorial team as well as the production teams at Beyond Words and Simon & Schuster, particularly Brianne Bardusch, Bailey Potter, Lindsay Easterbrooks-Brown, and Jennifer Weaver-Neist: thank you for your endless efforts, patience, and faith as we focused on the big vision of the project. Thank you to my self-care team, including my doctors, wellness experts, and medical-intuitive friends who supported my health journey and recovery: you helped me to heal myself as I learned firsthand the power of the process shared in this book.

Thank you to my rescue service dog, Chance, my very own Earth angel. While writing this book, we experienced back-to-back devasting traumas, but with the love in our hearts, we rose above even stronger, healthier, and happier than ever before. Thank you to my family—Clint, Rhonda, Mom, and Dad—for being in my inner circle and my best friends.

Thank you to God, my spirit team, angels, Summer Bacon and Dr. Peebles, Angelena, my ancestors, my higher self, and the entire collective of light workers bringing more love into the world. And from my heart to yours, dear reader, and to my beautiful coaching clients, and social media community, and the people who donated to the GoFundMe effort to "Help 'Chance' the Rescue, Service-Dog Walk Again." Your outpouring of love, generosity, and support helped us in a time of great need, showing us the true power of love and support. Forever grateful to you all.

To you, dear reader, thank you for showing up for yourself by choosing to prioritize your health, happiness, and wellness routine. May you experience excellent sleep every night and awaken every morning even more connected to your true self, your vibrancy, and the freedom to live your best days forward.

NOTES

1. "The State of Sleep Health in America 2023," America Sleep Apnea Association, accessed May 10, 2024, https://www.sleephealth.org/sleep-health/the-state-of-sleephealth-in-america/.

2. Vanessa Ling, "Sleep Apnea Statistics and Facts You Should Know," National Council on Aging, October 9, 2024, https://www.ncoa.org/adviser/sleep/sleep-apnea-statistics/.

3. Nicholas M. Hobson et al., "The Psychology of Rituals: An Integrative Review and Process-Based Framework," *Personality and Social Psychology Review* 22, no. 3 (August 2018): 260–84, https://doi.org/10.1177/1088868317734944.

4. "The State of Sleep Health in America 2023," American Sleep Apnea Association.

5. Phillip Huyett and Neil Bhattacharyya, "Incremental Health Care Utilization and Expenditures for Sleep Disorders in the United States," *Journal of Clinical Sleep Medicine* 17, no. 10 (October 1, 2021): 1981–86, https://doi.org/10.5664/jcsm.9392.

6. "The State of Sleep Health in America 2023," American Sleep Apnea Association.

7. Patricia Cernadas Curotto, Virginie Sterpenich, David Sander, Nicolas Favez, Ulrike Rimmele, and Olga Klimecki, "Quarreling After a Sleepless Night: Preliminary Evidence of the Impact of Sleep

Deprivation on Interpersonal Conflict," *Affective Science* 3, no. 2 (2022): 341–52, https://doi.org /10.1007/s42761-021-00076-4.

8. Institute of Medicine, "Extent and Health Consequences of Chronic Sleep Loss and Sleep Disorders" in *Sleep Disorders and Sleep Deprivation: An Unmet Public Health Problem*, ed. Harvey R. Colten and Bruce M. Altevogt (The National Academies Press, 2006): 55–136, https://nap.nationalacademies .org/read/11617/chapter/5.

9. "Sleep Deprivation and Deficiency," National Heart, Lung, and Blood Institute, last modified March 24, 2022, https://www.nhlbi.nih.gov/health-topics/sleep -deprivation-and-deficiency.

10. Brianna Graham, "One-Third of Us Lose Sleep to the 'Sunday Scaries.' Here's How to Get It Back," Sleep Foundation, last modified September 21, 2022, https://www.sleepfoundation.org/sleep-news/one -third-of-adults-lose-sleep-to-sunday-scaries.

11. Lisa Marie Basile, "Painsomnia Steals 51.5 Minutes of Our Sleep Every Night. How Do We Cope?" Sleep Foundation, last modified December 16, 2022, https://www.sleepfoundation.org/sleep-news /painsomnia-steals-an-hour-of-sleep-nightly.

12. "The State of Sleep Health in America 2023," American Sleep Apnea Association.

13. "Sleep Survey Results," RestoreZ, May 22, 2020, https://www.restorez.com/blogs/blog/sleep-survey -results.

14. Michael J. Maker, Simon A. Rego, and Gregory M. Asnis, "Sleep Disturbances in Patients with Post-Traumatic Stress Disorder: Epidemiology, Impact and Approaches to Management," *CNS Drugs* 20, no. 7 (July 2006): 567–90, https://doi.org/10.2165 /00023210-200620070-00003.

15. Marco Hafner et al., "Why Sleep Matters—the Economic Costs of Insufficient Sleep: A Cross-Country Comparative Analysis," *RAND Health Quarterly* 6, no. 4 (January 1, 2017): 11, https://www .ncbi.nlm.nih.gov/pmc/articles/PMC5627640/.

16. Laura Rubin, "Bedtime Rituals to Help You Sleep," last modified January 17, 2024, https://sleepdoctor .com/sleep-hygiene/bedtime-rituals/; Nicholas M. Hobson, Devin Bonk, and Michael Inzlicht, "Rituals Decrease the Neural Response to Performance Failure," *PeerJ* 5 (May 30, 2017), https://doi.org /10.7717/peerj.3363.

17. Jingyi Sun et al., "Sleep Deprivation and Gut Microbiota Dysbiosis: Current Understandings and Implications," International Journal of Molecular Sciences 24, no. 4 (May 31, 2023), 9603, https:// www.ncbi.nlm.nih.gov/pmc/articles/PMC10253795/; Katharine C. Simon, Lynn Nadel, and Jessica D. Payne, "The Functions of Sleep: A Cognitive Neuroscience Perspective," *PNAS* 119, no. 44 (October 24, 2022), https://www.ncbi.nlm.nih.gov/pmc/articles /PMC9636951/.

18. Matthew Walker, *Why We Sleep: Unlocking the Power of Sleep and Dreams* (Scribner, 2017), 7.

19. "Sleep and Mood," Division of Sleep Medicine, Harvard Medical School, last modified October 1, 2021, https://sleep.hms.harvard.edu/education -training/public-education/sleep-and-health-education -program/sleep-health-education-87; Eric Suni and Alex Dimitriu, "Stress and Insomnia," Sleep Foundation, last modified November 16, 2023, https://www.sleepfoundation.org/insomnia/stress -and-insomnia.

20. Christopher E. Kline, "The Bidirectional Relationship between Exercise and Sleep: Implications for Exercise Adherence and Sleep Improvement," *American Journal of Lifestyle Medicine* 8, no. 6. (November/December 2014): 375–79, https://journals.sagepub.com/doi/10 .1177/1559827614544437.

21. Danielle Pacheco and Anis Rehman, "Sleep Latency," Sleep Foundation, last modified January 18, 2023, https://www.sleepfoundation.org/how-sleep-works /sleep-latency.

22. WebMD Editorial Contributors, "Waking Up in the Middle of the Night," WebMD, last modified February 21, 2022, https://www.webmd.com/sleep -disorders/stay-asleep.

23. Susan Moran, "The Science behind Finding Your Mantra—and How to Practice It Daily," *Yoga Journal*, last modified February 3, 2022, https://www.yoga

journal.com/yoga-101/sanskrit/mantras-101-the-science
-behind-finding-your-mantra-and-how-to-practice-it/.

24. Abhimanyu Ganguly et al., "Effect of Meditation
on Autonomic Function in Healthy Individuals:
A Longitudinal Study," *Journal of Family Medicine
and Primary Care* 9, no. 8 (August 2020): 3944–48,
https://doi.org/10.4103/jfmpc.jfmpc_460_20.

25. Heather L. Rusch et al., "The Effect of Mindfulness
Meditation on Sleep Quality: A Systematic Review
and Meta-Analysis of Randomized Controlled Trials,"
Annals of the New York Academy of Sciences 1445, no. 1
(June 2019): 5–16, https://doi.org/10.1111/nyas.13996.

26. Katherine R. Arlinghaus and Craig A. Johnston,
"The Importance of Creating Habits and Routine,"
American Journal of Lifestyle Medicine 13, no. 2
(March/April 2019): 142–44, https://doi.org/10.1177
/1559827618818044.

27. Marcia P. Jimenez et al., "Associations between Nature
Exposure and Health: A Review of the Evidence,"
*International Journal of Environmental Research and
Public Health* 18, no. 9 (2021): 4790, https://doi
.org/10.3390/ijerph18094790.

28. Andrew Huberman, "Using Light for Health,"
Huberman Lab, January 24, 2023, https://www
.hubermanlab.com/newsletter/using-light-for-health.

29. Marius Marici et al., "Is Rejection, Parental
Abandonment or Neglect a Trigger for Higher
Perceived Shame and Guilt in Adolescents?"

Healthcare 11, no. 12 (June 12, 2023): 1724, https:// www.ncbi.nlm.nih.gov/pmc/articles/PMC10298591/.

30. Mary-Frances O'Connor and Saren H. Seeley, "Grieving as a Form of Learning: Insights from Neuroscience Applied to Grief and Loss," *Current Opinion in Psychology* 43 (February 2022): 317–22, https://doi.org/10.1016/j.copsyc.2021.08.019.

31. Kiara Anthony, "EFT Tapping," Heathline, last modified April 6, 2023, https://www.healthline.com /health/eft-tapping#technique.

32. Deepak Langade et al., "Efficacy and Safety of Ashwagandha (Withania somnifera) Root Extract in Insomnia and Anxiety: A Double-Blind, Randomized, Placebo-Controlled Study," *Cureus* 11, no. 9 (September 28, 2019), https://doi.org/10.7759/cureus.5797.

33. Karen O'Donnell, "How PTSD Treatment Can Learn from Ancient Warrior Rituals," The Conversation, November 30, 2016, https://theconversation.com /how-ptsd-treatment-can-learn-from-ancient-warrior -rituals-69589.

34. James L. Oschman, Gaétan Chevalier, and Richard Brown, "The Effects of Grounding (Earthing) on Inflammation, Wound Healing, and Prevention and Treatment of Chronic Inflammatory and Autoimmune Diseases," *Journal of Inflammation Research* 2015, no. 8 (March 24, 2015): 83–96, https://doi.org/10.2147/JIR.S69656.

35. Julie Ober Allen et al., "Experiences of Everyday Ageism and the Health of Older US Adults," *JAMA*

Network Open 5, no. 6 (June 15, 2022), https://www
.ncbi.nlm.nih.gov/pmc/articles/PMC9201677/.

36. César Fernández-de-las-Peñas et al., "Sleep
    Disturbances in Tension-Type Headache and
    Migraine," *Therapeutic Advances in Neurological
    Disorders* 11 (2018), https://doi.org/10.1177
    /1756285617745444.

37. Hedy Marks, "Sleep Deprivation and Memory Loss,"
    WebMD, August 2, 2022, https://www.webmd.com
    /sleep-disorders/sleep-deprivation-effects-on-memory.

38. Hyun Jeong Han et al., "Effects of Red Ginseng
    Extract on Sleeping Behaviors in Human Volunteers,"
    Journal of Ethnopharmacology 149, no. 2 (September
    16, 2013): 597–99, https://doi.org/10.1016/j.jep
    .2013.07.005.

39. Nicole Lovato and Leon Lack, "The Effects of
    Napping on Cognitive Functioning," *Progress in Brain
    Research* 185 (2010): 155–66, https://doi.org/10.1016
    /B978-0-444-53702-7.00009-9.

40. Adam Rowden, "What to Know about Amygdala
    Hijack," Medical News Today, April 19, 2021, https://
    www.medicalnewstoday.com/articles/amygdala-hijack.

41. Brant P. Hasler and Anne Germain, "Correlates and
    Treatments of Nightmares in Adults," *Sleep Medicine
    Clinics* 4, no. 4 (December 2009): 507–17, https://
    doi.org/10.1016/j.jsmc.2009.07.012; Rob Newsom
    and Alex Dimitriu, "How Trauma Affects Dreams,"
    Sleep Foundation, January 3, 2024, https://www

.sleepfoundation.org/dreams/how-trauma-can-affect
-dreams.

42. Matthew R Ebben, Peter Yan, and Ana C. Krieger,
"The Effects of White Noise on Sleep and Duration in
Individuals Living in a High Noise Environment
in New York City," *Sleep Medicine* 83, (July 2021):
256–59, https://www.sciencedirect.com/science
/article/abs/pii/S1389945721002021.

43. Kendra Cherry, "How Cognitive Biases Influence
the Way You Think and Act," Verywell Mind, last
modified May 7, 2024, https://www.verywellmind
.com/what-is-a-cognitive-bias-2794963.

44. Majd A. Alnawwar et al., "The Effect of Physical
Activity on Sleep Quality and Sleep Disorder: A
Systematic Review," *Cureus* 15, no. 8 (August 16,
2023), https://doi.org/10.7759/cureus.43595.

45. Janne Tuomi, Minna Kuurne-Koivisto, and Markku
Partinen, "The Effects of Whole-Body Vibration
Therapy on Patients with Primary Insomnia,"
University of Helsinki, 2016, https://helda.helsinki.fi
/items/6e08898a-8e7d-42be-bbfa-7b9436db187d.

46. Eric Suni and Dustin Cotliar, "How to Fix Your Sleep
Schedule," Sleep Foundation, last modified December
8, 2023, https://www.sleepfoundation.org/sleep
-hygiene/how-to-reset-your-sleep-routine.

47. Noriko Shinjyo, Guy Waddell, and Julia Green,
"Valerian Root in Treating Sleep Problems and
Associated Disorders—a Systematic Review and
Meta-Analysis," *Journal of Evidence-Based Integrated*

Medicine 25 (2020), https://doi.org/10.1177
/2515690X20967323.

48. Nancy A. Curry and Tim Kasser, "Can Coloring Mandalas Reduce Anxiety?" *Art Therapy* 22, no. 2 (2005): 81–85, https://doi.org/10.1080/07421656 .2005.10129441.

49. Scott Barry Kaufman et al., "The Light vs. Dark Triad of Personality: Contrasting Two Very Different Profiles of Human Nature," *Frontiers in Psychology* 10 (March 11, 2019): 467, https://doi.org/10.3389 /fpsyg.2019.00467; Taylor J. Vossen et al., "Exploring the Dark Side: Relationships between the Dark Triad Traits and Cluster B Personality Disorder Features," *Journal of Psychiatry and Psychiatric Disorders* 1, no. 6 (October 23, 2017): 317–26, https://www.fortune journals.com/articles/exploring-the-dark-side -relationships-between-the-dark-triad-traits-and -cluster-b-personality-disorder-features.html.

50. "Highly Sensitive Person," *Psychology Today*, accessed June 24, 2024, https://www.psychologytoday.com/us /basics/highly-sensitive-person.

51. Yufang Lin, "Your Vagus Nerve May Be Key To Fighting Anxiety and Stress," interview by Cleveland Clinic, April 20, 2023, https://health.clevelandclinic .org/what-does-the-vagus-nerve-do.

52. Iris Waichler, "Post-Traumatic Growth (PTG): What It Looks Like & How to Begin," Choosing Therapy, May 7, 2024, https://www.choosingtherapy.com /post-traumatic-growth/.

53. E. Stobbe et al., "Birdsongs Alleviate Anxiety and Paranoia in Healthy Participants," *Scientific Reports* 12 (October 13, 2022), https://doi.org/10.1038/s41598 -022-20841-0.

54. Stefanie Valentic, "More Than Half of Americans Have Unhealthy Work-Life Balance," *EHS Today*, May 2, 2019, https://www.ehstoday.com/health/article /21920133/more-than-half-of-americans-have -unhealthy-work-life-balance.

55. Heidi Godman, "Having a Hobby Tied to Happiness and Well-Being," Harvard Health Publishing, January 1, 2024, https://www.health.harvard.edu/mind-and -mood/having-a-hobby-tied-to-happiness-and -well-being.

56. Tracy Brandmeyer and Arnaud Delorme, "Meditation and the Wandering Mind: A Theoretical Framework of Underlying Neurocognitive Mechanisms," *Perspectives on Psychological Science* 16, no. 1 (January 2021): 39–66, https://doi.org/10.1177/17456916209 17340.

57. Raminder Mulla, "Can't Sleep? Overthinking? How Thought Blocking Can Help," Sleepstation, last modified December 6, 2021, https://www.sleepstation .org.uk/articles/sleep-tips/thought-blocking/.

58. John Gravois, "You're Not Fooling Anyone," *Chronicle of Higher Education*, November 9, 2007, https://www .chronicle.com/article/youre-not-fooling-anyone/.

59. Robert Pepperell, "Consciousness as a Physical Process Caused by the Organization of Energy in the Brain,"

Frontiers in Psychology 9 (November 1, 2018), https://doi.org/10.3389/fpsyg.2018.02091.

60. "The Famous Ho'oponopono Words of the 4-Phrase Hawaiian Forgiveness Mantra," Ho'oponopono Miracle, accessed June 25, 2024, https://hooponoponomiracle.com/iloveyou-imsorry-pleaseforgiveme-thankyou-mantra/.

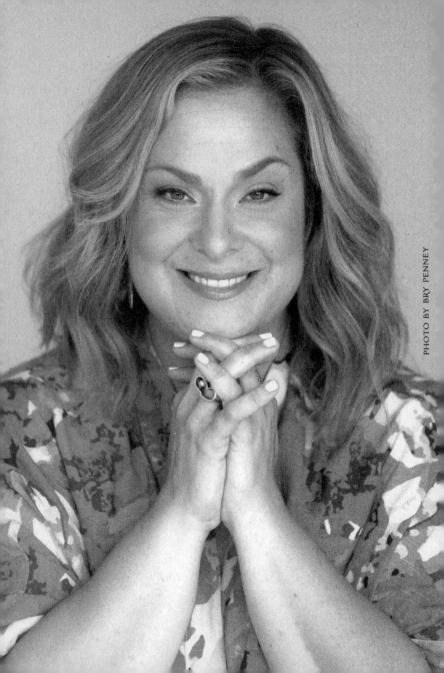

ABOUT THE AUTHOR

Shannon Kaiser is a world-renowned spiritual and self-love teacher, speaker, and acclaimed empowerment coach; a bestselling author of seven books on the psychology of happiness and fulfillment including *The Self-Love Experiment*, named number one of the "20 Self-Love Books That Will Lift You Up" by *Oprah* magazine; and the designer and creator of two mantra decks and two oracle decks. She guides people to awaken and align to their true selves so they can live their highest potential. Shannon's signature teaching is transformative, bridging spiritual and ancient wisdom with modern practical wisdom. Her self-inquiry and personal transformation books, programs, social media channels, and viral reels have reached 22 million people a month. She's been named among the "Top 100 Women to Watch in Wellness" by mindbodygreen, "your go-to happiness booster" by Health magazine, and "one of the freshest voices in mental health and wellness" by *Chicken Soup for the Woman's Soul*. Connect with her on social media @ ShannonKaiserWrites and her websites PlayWithTheWorld .com and RadicalBodyLovewithShannon.com.

Books and Card Decks
by Shannon Kaiser

Brought to you by Beyond Words Publishing

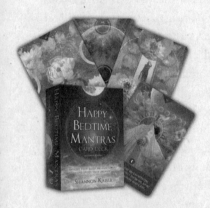

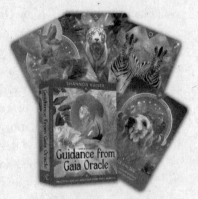

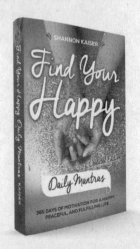

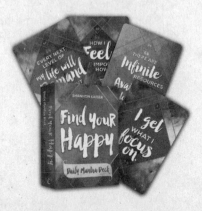